D1117902

Essential
Mental Health
Nursing Skills

Commissioning Editor: Ninette Premdas
Development Editors: Mairi McCubbin, Fiona Conn
Project Manager: Jess Thompson
Design Direction: Judith Wright
Illustrator: Barking Dog Art
Illustration Manager: Gillian Richards

Essential Mental Health Nursing Skills

Madeline O'Carroll MSc PGDip(HE) RMN RGN

Lecturer, St Bartholomew School of Nursing, City University, London, UK

Alistair Park MSc PGDip(Ed) RMN RNT

Lecturer, St Bartholomew School of Nursing, City University, London, UK

Series Editor

Maggie Nicol BSc(Hons) MSc PGDip(Ed) RGN

Professor of Clinical Skills, St Bartholomew School of Nursing, City University, London, UK

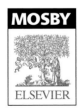

Edinburgh London New York Oxford Philadelphia St Louis Sydney Toronto 2007

MOSBY
ELSEVIER

An imprint of Elsevier Limited

First published 2007

ISBN 978-0-7234-3348-4

British Library Cataloguing in Publication Data
A catalogue record for this book is available from the British Library

Library of Congress Cataloging in Publication Data
A catalog record for this book is available from the Library of Congress

Notice
Neither the Publisher nor the authors assume any responsibility for any loss or injury and/or damage to persons or property arising out of or related to any use of the material contained in this book. It is the responsibility of the treating practitioner, relying on independent expertise and knowledge of the patient, to determine the best treatment and method of application for the patient.

The Publisher

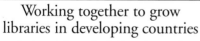

Working together to grow
libraries in developing countries

www.elsevier.com | www.bookaid.org | www.sabre.org

ELSEVIER   BOOK AID International   Sabre Foundation

ELSEVIER   your source for books, journals and multimedia in the health sciences
www.elsevierhealth.com

The publisher's policy is to use paper manufactured from sustainable forests

Printed in China

Contents

Preface

WHY THIS BOOK?

This book is a practical guide to developing the skills essential for mental health nursing in the twenty-first century. It aims to provide an easily comprehensible structure for understanding the essential aspects of mental health nursing and their application in practice.

Contemporary mental health nursing is a complex matrix of theoretical concepts, models, frameworks, competencies and policies. This barrage of ideas and perspectives can seem bewildering for a student nurse trying to learn his or her role in practice. The aim of this book is to help the student develop the skills needed for the practice environment. It identifies the skills essential for the mental health nurse and provides an easy to understand guide to 'what to do and how to do it'. The book draws on the policy and theoretical underpinnings of mental health nursing but concentrates on the essential skills and their application in practice.

WHAT IT IS

The book identifies the four essential skills that we believe are fundamental to the practice of mental health nursing. These skills can be used with different patients and service users and transferred, like a toolkit, between the many settings and services with which mental health nurses today are involved.

The book is organized into two sections. After outlining the background to contemporary mental health nursing in Chapter 1, the first identifies the four essential skills. These are the ability to form therapeutic relationships, observation, taking on different roles and reflection. The second section concentrates on the process of care and provides the context in which the essential skills are applied. It covers communication, assessment, care delivery, improving physical well-being and managing care. The chapter on improving physical well-being is supported with an appendix that describes the clinical observation skills that are used to assess physical health.

The focus is on developing the student's ability to use the skills in the practice environment. Some background perspective to each skill is provided, followed by an easily understandable outline of the main points for practice. Examples demonstrating how the skills can be applied across the diversity found in modern mental health nursing are included.

HOW DO I USE IT?

This book provides an easy to understand and practical framework for the development and use of the skills essential to mental health nursing. It is designed to be taken with you to the practice environment so that you can easily refer to it when you are learning a skill. You should always be supervised by a registered nurse until you are competent at a particular skill.

Many of the skills are based on things we do naturally, such as observation and assessment. We start by asking you to think about how you currently use these skills and show how they can be adapted and developed for nursing practice. Each chapter includes an introduction to the skill or application with a small amount of theoretical background, and is then divided into sections concentrating on the key issues for practice. Examples from practice are included to help illustrate the material but you are encouraged to use the activity boxes provided throughout the book to explore an area using examples from your own experience.

We hope that you will enjoy reading the book and find it useful during your career in mental health nursing.

Madeline O'Carroll and Alistair Park, 2007

1

The essence of mental health nursing

In this job you're often working with people when they're at their lowest point and that can be very demanding. But the other side is that when you see people recovering and you feel that you've been part of making that happen it's immensely rewarding.

Charge nurse

INTRODUCTION

Mental health nursing is about working with people, often when they are at their most distressed. Mental health practice is informed by knowledge and attitudes which shape the skills that are used in interactions between nurses and patients and service users. The twenty-first century is an exciting time to be a mental health nurse; the UK government has made mental health one of its priorities, and this has resulted in significant financial input. Perhaps equally important is the number of documents that have been published (e.g. *Review of Mental Health Nursing*, *National Service Framework for Mental Health* and *Mental Health Policy Implementation Guidelines*), which represent considerable thinking about mental health nursing, policy and service organization. The most significant element of these documents reflects a real shift in the relations between people using mental health services and mental health nurses and other professionals. There is now an expectation that nurses will work in partnership with people using mental health services and their families, rather than expecting them to be passive recipients of care. This will require changes to education, training and service organization in order for this to happen.

In order to move forward, it is important to understand the past as this has a strong influence, especially in defining nurses' identity and shaping services (Nolan 2000). This chapter outlines the origins of mental health care and the development of mental health nursing. We then move to the current context and identify some of the key policy documents that are influencing practice. Effective mental health nursing is underpinned by attitudes and beliefs that reflect contemporary knowledge about mental health and mental illness, and we explore these. Finally, we explain the structure of the book and the thinking behind the two sections.

ORIGINS OF MENTAL HEALTH CARE IN EUROPE

The concept of mental health care is a relatively recent one and, in western societies, it emerged with the shift towards an individualistic perspective. Before this time, ideas about health and well-being came from the communities in which people lived. Codes of behaviour were developed and passed between the generations, and this included rules about how emotions should be both experienced and managed. For example, following the death of a loved one, acceptable reactions in different communities might range from loud weeping and wailing to quiet crying or withholding any expression of emotion. Early texts indicate that there has always been a minority of people whose experiences were recognized as being stronger than others. Sometimes, this took the form of melancholia (this would now be called depression) or visions and, in some cultures, these phenomena, and the people who experienced them, were highly esteemed. Mostly, this group was part of the community although, occasionally, they were made to leave and became outcasts (Porter 2002).

In Europe, Christianity was the source of religious beliefs, moral guidance and the development of a form of social welfare. The Catholic Church in England had an extensive network of monasteries through which it provided care and asylum when families or communities were unable to take on these duties. The dissolution of the monasteries in the sixteenth century brought this to an abrupt end. Into this vacuum soon emerged the figure of 'poor Tom', as described in Shakespeare's *King Lear*. This represented, if not a real person, at least the idea of a man driven to madness and left to wander the country as a beggar as there was no longer a place where he might be cared for and contained.

From the seventeenth century onwards, private 'mad houses' were established for those with the means to pay. Care is thought to have been variable and, at times, downright cruel by modern standards. The Retreat at York, established in 1794, was founded on Quaker principles and marked a change in attitude to the care of the mentally ill (Nolan 1993). In some respects, it was also a return to an earlier time when spiritual beliefs informed attitudes.

The birth of the mental health nurse

The next major shift in caring for people with mental illness took place in the middle of the nineteenth century. This came in the wake of rapid industrialization, which resulted in enormous social upheaval as thousands left the land and flocked to the new industrial cities to work. This resulted in the age of the asylum: vast self-contained institutions housing patients and staff. In the development of mental health nursing, this is really the birthplace of the 'mental nurse': men and women whose early origins were quite different from those of the (female) general nurse.

Initially, there was no training for the doctors or nurses who worked in the asylums. The first record of training for nurses was a series of lectures organized by the Medical Superintendent at the Royal Edinburgh Asylum in 1854. This eventually led to the publication of a handbook for attendants and, later, a formal training. To some extent, the asylums provided a laboratory for the development of psychiatry, at this time a new branch of medicine. Staff titles also reflected this development as staff who were originally called 'lunatic attendants' gradually became 'mental nurses' and later 'psychiatric nurses'.

By the middle of the twentieth century, a number of factors combined to contribute to the demise of the Victorian mental hospital as representing the pinnacle of mental health care. A number of different models began to emerge including an alternative to hospital in the form of community-based care (de-institutionalization). The 'anti-psychiatry' movement, represented in part by the writing of Laing (see Laing & Esterson 1964) and Szasz (1961) also proposed new ways of understanding both mental illness and how it should be treated. Medication such as chlorpromazine was also being developed, which could be used to treat the symptoms of psychosis. One of the most powerful factors behind the reforms was the sheer cost of the asylum system, which became unaffordable in a postwar period that saw the introduction of the welfare state.

De-institutionalization

The policy of de-institutionalization impacted on nurses as well as those for whom they cared. Many nurses also moved into the community and, like their patients, they were not always sufficiently well supported to manage this transition. Gradually, training became available for nurses taking up roles outside the hospital with the development of courses for community psychiatric nurses. As well as taking on more specialized roles, the notion of the nurse as therapist also emerged with the advent of the behavioural nurse therapist, an early example of an evidence-based approach to care.

Changes in nurse education

As the large asylums were no longer seen as the preferred place for the care and treatment of patients, by the middle of the 1980s, hospitals were no longer deemed to be the ideal location for nurse education. The Project 2000 initiative (UKCC 1986) saw a move away from hospital-based training into higher education. This also meant a significant shift for mental health nurses to the current system of shared training with nurses from other branches through a common foundation programme. Initially, the foundation programme lasted for 18 months, but the training was criticized for its inability to produce nurses 'fit to practise'. Consequently, the foundation programme has been reduced to 1 year, and the branch part of the programme has been increased to 2 years (UKCC 1999).

There is plenty of scope for the development of mental health nursing within higher education. For example, there are opportunities for interprofessional training and education that are only beginning to be explored. Even less developed are ideas about how to use the experience and expertise of service users in this context.

Review of mental health nursing

In 2005, the Chief Nursing Officer (CNO) of England set up a review to address the question: 'How can mental health nursing best contribute to the care of service users in the future?' (Department of Health 2006). The review process began with an extensive consultation that included service users, nurses and other mental health professionals and organizations. It also included a literature review that covered the following areas:

- the efficacy of mental health nursing interventions
- service users' and carers' views of mental health nursing
- stress and mental health nursing/recruitment and retention.

The review identified a number of recommendations that were grouped into three broad themes which reflected the vision for mental health nursing over the next 10 years. Examples of good practice are also included in the review.

Putting values into practice

The CNO acknowledged that the values and attitudes held by nurses have a significant impact on the care they deliver. The review identified three key 'values' that need to be incorporated into practice: recovery, equality and evidence-based practice. The recovery approach is not just about working actively with service users to assist them to identify and achieve their goals. It is clear that social exclusion has a negative effect on outcome and needs to be addressed. Staff also need to adopt more optimistic attitudes towards the ability of patients and service users to change.

There is evidence that some people fail to receive adequate health care or may experience discrimination on account of factors including age, race and sexuality. Nurses need to actively evaluate the care they deliver as well as influencing the development of services that are more able to manage difference.

The final area in this section is basing practice on best evidence. It is worth noting that the report urges nurses to draw on a range of types of evidence including the views of service users and carers.

Improving outcomes

This section identifies who should be receiving care and the type of care that nurses should deliver. Although nurses are the largest professional group in mental health, they are nonetheless a limited resource and therefore need to target their services carefully. The review recommends that mental health nurses focus on those with complex difficulties and higher levels of need. A number of new roles have been developed in mental health such as graduate mental health workers who are not allied to any professional group. Mental health nurses are well placed to support these workers as they deal with individuals (usually in primary care) who have less complex needs.

Interpersonal relationships with service users and carers are central to mental health nursing and impact on all aspects of care. Nurses should make assessments that incorporate psychological, social, physical and spiritual needs as well as being able to assess and manage risk. It is also important to assess an individual's strengths and abilities.

The review recommends that nurses need to be more involved with improving the physical well-being of people with mental health problems. Specific areas of practice that are highlighted are the need to respond to people with substance misuse problems and improve inpatient care.

A positive, modern profession

The final section addresses the multidisciplinary context in which nurses work and also considers what needs to be done to implement the proposed changes. Nursing has already developed new roles (e.g. modern matron, nurse consultant) as well as working in new services such as prison in-reach and home treatment teams. New roles will continue to be necessary, but it is important that they are able to improve service user outcomes.

This section also identifies difficulties experienced by some mental health nurses. This includes problems expressing themselves assertively, particularly within multidisciplinary teams. The literature review conducted as part of the CNO's review identified the fact that mental health nursing can be stressful. Therefore, consideration must be given to strategies for recruiting and retaining staff. Education at pre- and post-registration level has a vital role to play.

Generally, responses to the review have been favourable. The Sainsbury Centre for Mental Health (SCMH 2006) supports the recommendations, but finds the review 'too cautious' and wonders how some changes will be possible in the absence of additional funding.

Changes to mental health services

It is difficult to separate patterns of health care from the social context from which they arise. When an individual is identified as needing care, whether the care is in a monastery, an asylum or their own home, the treatment they receive will depend on the relative benevolence of those providing the care. In recent years, there have been changes in the relationships between people using mental health services and the staff providing them that have occurred as a result of broader social changes. From the 1980s onwards, there has been a move towards economic liberalization in many developed countries including the UK and the USA. This has included rescinding legislation that hampered trade and economic markets, reducing the power of the professionals as well as encouraging the growth of the consumer. In the UK, a number of reforms were introduced into the health service including a split between those providing health care and the health authorities who purchase it. One of the criticisms of the many changes that were introduced during this time is that they failed to impact on the actual face-to-face care that patients received (Onyett 2004).

At the same time, the voice of the mental health service user was growing increasingly loud. Some viewed services as being so toxic that they called themselves survivors of the psychiatric system. Again, this was part of a wider movement of people who saw themselves as being socially excluded, disadvantaged and discriminated against, and who decided that the time had come for major changes.

From patient to service user

These shifts have also been reflected in the language used to represent the person receiving health care. Language is particularly interesting for what it can reveal about underlying attitudes and beliefs. In the past, people experiencing mental distress were variously described as lunatics or mad men or women. Under the asylum system, the idea of being a patient was introduced; initially, people were called mental patients, although this gradually changed to psychiatric patient. A current term is mental health patient (no one is called a mental illness patient). The term client is also used, generally in relation to people served by community services. More recently, the term 'service user' is increasingly being used. It seems to reflect an element of the person opting into or taking up services, and suggests a more active engagement than that represented by the word 'patient'. In this text, we use the terms patient and service user as they seem to represent different facets of the experience of the person with a mental health problem.

MENTAL HEALTH POLICY IN THE TWENTY-FIRST CENTURY

Having considered some of the factors influencing the development of mental health care and nursing, it is important to identify the issues pertinent to contemporary practice. In the UK, mental health, along with cancer and heart disease, has been identified as one of three health priorities by the government (Department of Health 1999a). As a result, a number of policy documents and reports have been produced with the aim of modernizing twenty-first century mental health services. Initial work produced a *National Service Framework* (NSF) *for Mental Health* (Department of Health 1999b), which addressed the mental health needs of adults and set out standards and service models. *National Service Frameworks for Older People* (Department of Health 2001) and *Children* (Department of Health 2004a) have also been produced. In 2004, the National Director for Mental Health reported on the first 5 years of the NSF and outlined his vision for the next 5 years, which included more patient choice, the care of long-term conditions and improved access to services (Department of Health 2004b).

Attention has also been given to the type of practitioners required to provide these services, and a number of documents have been published. The key documents are: *The Capable Practitioner* produced by the Sainsbury Centre for Mental Health (SCMH 2000), *The National Occupational Standards for Mental Health* (www.skillsforhealth.org.uk/mentalhealth/) and, more recently, *The Ten Essential Shared Capabilities; A Framework for the Whole of the Mental Health Workforce* (Department of Health 2004c).

The Capable Practitioner

The Capable Practitioner (SCMH 2000) acknowledges both the fundamental changes happening in the mental health arena and the speed with which this has happened. In part, these changes relate to the move from hospital to community care that has been under way for a number of decades, but also recognize that services are becoming increasingly specialized and complex. For example, initiatives such as 'assertive outreach' and 'home treatment teams' hardly existed a decade ago, at least not outside research initiatives. Now, they are expected to be part of general service provision. Another major shift relates to the range of agencies (health, social services and the voluntary sector) now involved in delivering care. Education and training also make an important contribution to the care and recovery of people with mental health problems. The challenge for staff is to find ways to work effectively with patients and carers and to liaise and negotiate with many different agencies.

The Capable Practitioner (SCMH 2000) set out to identify a broad framework of skills, knowledge and attitudes that would be appropriate for practitioners working in adult mental health services. The key areas are as follows.

Ethical practice

This refers to the values and attitudes that underpin the practice of mental health workers. In addition, professional workers such as nurses have their own codes of professional conduct (see Nursing and Midwifery Council 2004) and guidance for student nurses (see Nursing and Midwifery Council 2002, 2005). All these documents are essential reading for all mental health nurses and students.

Knowledge

'Knowledge is the foundation of effective practice' (SCMH 2000: 11). Here, this refers specifically to knowledge of policy and legislation as well as knowledge of mental health and mental health services. In order to provide effective services, it is necessary to draw on knowledge from a range of areas.

Process of care

Mental health care has become increasingly complex. Care is influenced by policy and legislation and may be delivered by a number of different agencies particularly health and social care. Therefore, co-ordination of care is essential. At the point of delivery, the process of care is about optimizing the relationship with service users and their carers as well as encouraging user participation. A range of capabilities is necessary for this including communication, assessment, care planning and supervision.

Interventions

The report states that practitioners must be able to deliver evidence-based interventions. Four categories of biopsychosocial and health promotional interventions are presented: medical and physical care interventions (e.g. medication management); psychological interventions (e.g. motivational interviewing); social and practical interventions such as support with housing and education; and mental health promotion that addresses social exclusion. These are all discussed in Chapter 8.

The National Occupational Standards for Mental Health

The National Occupational Standards for Mental Health (www.skillsforhealth. org.uk/mentalhealth/) were developed as part of a general move to produce a *Knowledge and Skills Framework for the National Health Service* (Department of Health 2004d) and to complement the work of *The Capable Practitioner* (SCMH 2000). *The National Occupational Standards for Mental Health* identify the purpose of mental health services as follows:

Work with individuals, families, groups, communities and agencies to provide equitable and non-discriminatory services, across all age groups and settings, which:

- promote mental health
- address mental health needs
- manage risk and
- provide appropriate support to people with mental health needs and their carers.

The Ten Essential Shared Capabilities

The document *The Ten Essential Shared Capabilities* (Department of Health 2004c) is the product of a collaboration between the National Health Service University (NHSU), the Sainsbury Centre for Mental Health and the National Institute for Mental Health in England (NIMHE), and links the work of *The Capable Practitioner* and the *Knowledge and Skills Framework* (Department of Health 2004d). Of particular importance is that it specifies what should be included in all training including pre-qualification training for professional staff (Box 1.1).

Key themes

The key themes that emerge from all three documents are: ethical practice, working in partnership and evidence-based practice, and an emphasis on

---

Box 1.1 The 10 essential shared capabilities: a framework for the whole of the mental health workforce

The 10 essential shared capabilities for mental health practice are:

Working in partnership
Respecting diversity
Practising ethically
Challenging inequality
Promoting recovery
Identifying people's needs and strengths
Providing service user-centred care
Making a difference
Promoting safety and positive risk-taking
Personal development and learning

---

mental health promotion. It can be argued that *The Ten Essential Shared Capabilities* aims to introduce some radical changes to practice with its inclusion of ideas such as promoting recovery and positive risk-taking. Recovery in this context is a concept that has its origins in service user approaches to working with psychosis. For staff, it requires attitudes that reflect a more hopeful and optimistic way of thinking about working with service users and assisting them to 'recover' what has been lost through illness. With the capability 'promoting safety and positive risk-taking', there is recognition of the tension between promoting safety and taking risks.

Attitudes and beliefs

Our ability to work in partnership is influenced by the attitudes and beliefs that we hold. It is important to be aware that our understanding of mental health and mental illness predates any training we may have undertaken; it is rooted in how our family and society explained and made sense of these concepts. For example, a commonly held belief is that people with mental health problems are in some way different from others, but psychological investigations have not been able to produce any evidence to support this view. In fact, research has shown that phenomena such as hallucinations (once thought to be only experienced by people who were mentally ill) are also common in people with no history of mental health problems.

When we make the decision to become a mental health nurse, it is extremely likely that we will hold some beliefs that do not reflect contemporary knowledge or attitudes. Therefore, it is important to develop a willingness and an ability to subject our beliefs to scrutiny rather than automatically acting as if they were true. One of the crucial differences between education and training is that education has the capacity to transform attitudes and beliefs. So, a university-based course provides an ideal forum for examining old and new knowledge as well as beliefs. We also have the tool of reflection (Chapter 5) to help us to review our practice to ensure that we operate within the ethical parameters expected by service users, the Nursing and Midwifery Council and other stakeholders.

A FRAMEWORK FOR MENTAL HEALTH NURSING

Although this book focuses on skills, these are not used in isolation; they need to be clearly situated within the context of contemporary practice. This requires mental health practitioners to think and reflect on their practice at all stages of their interactions with people, which means before making contact and during contact as well as following contact.

In this book, we present a simple framework that outlines the areas that need to be considered. These are policy, evidence, ethical aspects and skills (see Figure 1.1). To use this framework, you need to identify an area of practice, for example a service such as forensic or a home treatment team, or you might identify working with people with a specific diagnosis, for example personality disorder or dementia. Having identified your focus, you then need to consider each area in turn and use the information to inform your practice.

Policy and legislation

The first quadrant to consider is policy and legislation. Nurses should be familiar with the key documents such as the *National Service Framework for Mental Health* (Department of Health 1999b) that have already been described (see p. 8). Other policy documents include *Mental Health Policy Implementation Guidelines* (see www.dh.gov.uk/policyandguidance/mentalhealthpublications). These provide more detailed guidance on a range of areas including early intervention in psychosis, acute inpatient care and community mental health teams. The National Institute for Health and Clinical Excellence (NICE, formerly the National Institute for Clinical Excellence) also produces guide-

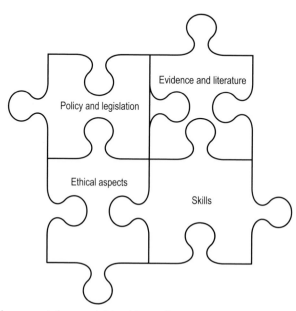

Figure 1.1 A framework for mental health nursing.

lines and recommendations regarding treatments and interventions for conditions including schizophrenia, depression, eating disorders and post-traumatic stress disorder. NICE has also produced guidance on the management of disturbed/violent behaviour. New documents are being produced all the time, and so it is important to keep up to date with current policy (see www.nice.org.uk).

In addition to national policy, most Mental Health Trusts and services also produce local guidelines that must be consulted. These may relate to a range of areas such as the administration of medication and policies regarding visiting patients at home. These are often located on the Trust intranet to ensure availability of the most recent version.

The majority of patients are admitted to hospital voluntarily and are referred to as 'informal' patients. However, there are occasions when someone may be admitted to hospital for assessment or treatment against his or her wishes. In these circumstances, patients are described as being admitted or detained formally or 'under a section' (of the Mental Health Act). As a student, you should be aware of whether a patient is formal or informal and familiarize yourself with the Mental Health Act (HMSO 1983).

Evidence and literature

There is a strong focus on the use of evidence-based interventions. Whenever nurses make an intervention, they should think about whether there is any evidence to support what they are doing. This might range from considering the use of a cognitive behavioural intervention with a person who is hearing voices to thinking about the role of empathy in the nurse–patient relationship. Databases such as the Cochrane Library provide such evidence, where it exists, as well as journals dedicated specifically to reporting on recent developments in the evidence base. The Cochrane Library is an electronic database that provides information on interventions in health care including systematic reviews (see www.nelh.nhs.uk/cochrane). Evidence has been graded according to the quality of the evidence, and the randomized controlled trial (RCT) is generally considered to be the gold standard (National Institute for Clinical Excellence 2002). Clearly, students and mental health nurses will need to develop skills in evaluating evidence and become aware of the arguments for and against different types of evidence.

In the grading scheme used by NICE, case studies, expert committee reports or opinions as well as the clinical experiences of respected authorities are all considered to be valid forms of evidence. This type of information is more likely to be found in the literature. Students need to become familiar with the main texts in their field as well as knowing how to conduct a literature search to locate material elsewhere. Websites are increasingly being used as a source of information. Again, it is important for students to be able to critically evaluate information produced in this domain and to be aware that information on web pages may not have been subjected to peer review.

Ethical aspects

In mental health contexts, there is an inherent power imbalance between staff and patients that is open to abuse. It is essential for practitioners to take responsibility for managing this through a commitment to ethical practice. Professional bodies such as the Nursing and Midwifery Council recognize this by setting out a Code of Professional Conduct (Nursing and Midwifery Council 2004). Mental Health Trusts may also have their own ethical codes or guidelines, and you will need to adhere to these.

As a student, you should start by identifying areas in which ethical issues may arise, for example consent to treatment, confidentiality and respect for difference. Gradually, you will see that ethics permeates *all* aspects of care, such as communication and assessment, and is not restricted to a few areas. Again, reflection is a critical tool for developing a deeper and more complex understanding of how ethical issues may be seen and managed in practice.

Skills

The final quadrant is skills. Having identified an area of practice, you then need to consider which types of interventions are supported by the evidence or the literature. For example, in relation to substance misuse, this might include motivational interviewing whereas, in relation to dementia, this might include coping with memory loss. The skills component involves breaking down the intervention by identifying which skills are necessary. All care needs to be based on good communication skills, particularly listening, but particular conditions or problems will require specific input. For example, when working with someone who has memory problems, it would be important for the nurse to present information clearly and to make specific reference to the time of day or mealtimes in order to help to cue the person in to their environment.

Using the framework for mental health nursing

It is possible to use this framework in a number of ways. At the beginning of your career in mental health nursing, you will probably be thinking 'How should I work with the patients and service users I meet?' The policy documents mentioned earlier all include information about this. In relation to the literature and evidence, you could find out what patients and service users say they want. Finally, you would have to think about what skills you would need to translate what you have read into practice. As noted above, learning how to become an effective listener would be a good place to start.

As you work with different people, you might become curious about their experiences as well as the skills you are learning. For example, in your lectures at university and in the practice areas, you will probably hear a lot about the importance of empathy. You could explore this using the framework by searching for literature on the topic as well as considering what skills might be necessary in order to demonstrate empathy.

ESSENTIAL MENTAL HEALTH NURSING SKILLS

In thinking about the work of the mental health nurse, we have made a number of assumptions that we would now like to make explicit. Most importantly, mental health nursing is an interpersonal process, taking place between the patient or service user and the nurse and involving carers and other professionals. In this respect, we share Ritter's (1997) view of the nurse as a mediator assisting the patient to manage the boundary between his or her internal world and the outside or external world. The nurse often has a pivotal role in mediating and managing the patient's care with other professionals, especially in inpatient settings, as well as liaising with other agencies.

Contemporary mental health practice tends to draw on a number of different theoretical models, as a sufficiently unified evidence base to inform all areas of practice does not currently exist. The nearest we have is a bio-psychosocial model that draws on biological, psychological and social explanations regarding the onset and maintenance of mental health problems. Despite its limitations, the biopsychosocial model allows a range of beliefs and approaches to be used, and we have used it to inform the text. It also reflects our personal training and experience in analytic, cognitive behavioural and systems-oriented approaches to understanding the human experience.

Consequently, we have organized this book around the direct or face-to-face components of the work. Good care must be based on contemporary knowledge and evidence and be informed by appropriate attitudes and values. It is recognized that good care also needs to be supported by effective administration and management, but this does not fall within the remit of this book.

Acquiring new skills

Acquiring new skills will be a fundamental part of your development as a mental health nurse. In this book, we describe a number of techniques to help you do this.

Building on existing skills

Many of the skills we describe are based on things we do naturally, including observation (Chapter 3), assessment (Chapter 6), taking on different roles (Chapter 4) and reflecting on what has happened to ourselves or other people (Chapter 5). Whenever possible, we start by asking you to think about how you are currently using these skills. It is usually easier to start to understand something you are already familiar with rather than learning about an area that is completely new. However, it is important to be clear that a personal context (e.g. friendship) is quite different from a professional context (i.e. mental health nursing). This means that, although there will be some ways in which we use the skills that are familiar, we must also be prepared to use them in ways that are quite different.

Keeping a journal

A key way of learning is to keep a personal journal. This can be used to record external material such as what you 'notice' (see Chapter 3) in your practice placements or other environments. You should also start becoming aware of your internal experiences such as thoughts and feelings and bodily sensations, for example a rapid heart rate related to anxiety, as these can be an important source of information about yourself and your reactions to others. Noting this internal and external material has a number of functions. It provides you with a record of your learning that enables you to monitor your own development over time. It will also help to deepen your knowledge and understanding of yourself and others. In addition, using a journal can help to develop reflection skills.

Activity boxes

Throughout the book, we use activity boxes. These are designed to help you explore an area by generating material of your own that is related to the chapter. In this way, it is possible to become more actively involved with the learning process. Activity boxes are identified by a pen logo.

STRUCTURE OF THE BOOK

This book is a practical guide to developing the skills essential for mental health nursing in the twenty-first century. The book is organized into two sections: first, the essential skills, followed by the process of care in section two. Neither is enough on its own; both are required to address all aspects of care.

Section one: the essential skills

The first section identifies four essential skills that we believe are fundamental to being a mental health nurse. These are the ability to form therapeutic relationships, observation, taking on different roles and reflection.

Therapeutic relationships

The therapeutic relationship is central to mental health nursing. This chapter explores the characteristics of relationships in general and then identifies the features of a therapeutic relationship. All relationships need attention in order to develop and move through different stages. For the nurse, this usually involves being more active at the beginning and gradually reducing their input as the patient recovers.

Observation

Chapter 3 examines the role of observation and the skills required to observe effectively. Nurses are constantly engaged in observation of themselves, others and the environment. So, observation involves noticing the patient and how they interact with their environment, but it also involves observation of oneself as a participant in the therapeutic relationship. It is only by observing oneself that it is possible to engage in a therapeutic relationship.

Taking on different roles

Chapter 4 discusses the different roles that you will adopt. As a student, your main role is to learn about mental health nursing by observing or participating in the delivery of care. In the mental health context, the three main roles are: delivering care, providing information and managing emotion.

Reflection

Reflection has become an essential learning tool for practice-based professions such as nursing. In Chapter 5, we discuss why reflection is so important and outline different approaches to reflection. Like the skill of observation, reflection requires us to be aware of ourselves and our reactions and also to describe what we notice in practice. However, it goes further, requiring us to think about what theories or knowledge may relate to what we have experienced and observed. Reflection also has the potential to help us develop new knowledge.

Section two: the process of care

The second section relates to the process of care and covers communication, assessment, interventions, promoting physical well-being and managing care. The heading 'process of care' is drawn from the document *The Capable Practitioner* (SCMH 2000), although we have added 'interventions' to this section.

The process of care relates to the focus (e.g. communication) or provides the context for the care being delivered (e.g. assessment), but all the essential skills need to be considered in each context.

For example, if the nurse's goal is to make an assessment with the patient, observation is vital as soon as contact is made as it may alter the goal; the patient might have an injury or a physical complaint that requires immediate attention. Or there might be physical needs such as hunger or thirst that would also take precedence over the nurse's goal of assessment. Awareness of these aspects as well as noticing the patient's psychological state will influence how the nurse begins the process of establishing a therapeutic relationship. As part of the assessment process, nurses also have to make decisions about what role they should adopt. For example, if the nurse observes that the patient is very anxious, then managing emotion (anxiety) may also be more important than continuing with the assessment process. In some respects, reflection is the key to managing all this information and being able to take decisions about what action to take and, later, reflecting on the actions that were taken.

Communication

Listening is one of the most important skills because it is through this that we learn about the experience of the other person. We convey that we are listening through our verbal and non-verbal communication. Active listening is not always easy, and there are times when it can be difficult to give our full attention. Recognizing some of the difficulties can help us to keep our focus. Chapter 6 considers the communication skills required in mental health nursing and ways that you can develop these.

Assessment

In Chapter 7, we present assessment as a process and outline factors that need to be considered such as the location where the assessment is taking place. We then identify three broad areas of assessment: strengths, physical and mental health and risk. In addition to knowing what to assess, it is important to think about how to assess, and we consider the use of tools and questionnaires and the interview format.

Care delivery and interventions

Modern mental health needs to have a broad focus that includes looking at the individual in the context of their family and social environment. In Chapter 8, we identify a range of care and interventions including medical and physical care, psychological interventions as well as social and practical interventions, and health promotion.

Improving physical well-being

The physical health and well-being of people with mental health problems have at times been overlooked, and these people have higher rates of morbidity and mortality than the general population. Chapter 9 discusses some of the reasons for this and identifies the main physical health problems. The assessment of physical health is described and supported with an appendix that presents the key clinical observations. The chapter concludes by identifying interventions to improve physical well-being including health promotion.

Managing care

As a student, you need to be able to manage the care that you deliver yourself, for example by evaluating its effectiveness. Although other staff will be responsible for managing care, the information you provide them with will influence the decision-making process. Chapter 10 will explore these issues and your role as a member of a team.

CONCLUSION

The book offers a framework for the development of clinical skills and is designed to complement other texts. It will not provide the answers to all the questions you may have, but it will help you develop the skills you need to work with patients and service users as well as carers and colleagues as part of a modern mental health workforce. We hope that you will enjoy reading the book and find it useful as you begin your career in mental health nursing.

References

Department of Health (1999a) *Our Healthier Nation.* London: Department of Health.

Department of Health (1999b) *National Service Framework for Mental Health.* London: Department of Health.

Department of Health (2001) *The National Service Framework for Older People.* London: Department of Health.

Department of Health (2004a) *National Service Framework for Children, Young People and Maternity Services.* London: Department of Health.

Department of Health (2004b) *The National Service Framework for Mental Health – Five Years On.* London: Department of Health.

Department of Health (2004c) *The Ten Essential Shared Capabilities. A Framework for the Whole of the Mental Health Workforce.* London: Department of Health.

Department of Health (2004d) *The NHS Knowledge and Skills Framework (NHS KSF) and the Development Review Process.* London: Department of Health.

Department of Health (2006) *From Values to Action: The Chief Nursing Officer's Review of Mental Health Nursing.* London: Department of Health.

HMSO (1983) Mental Health Act. London: HMSO.

Laing RD, Esterson A (1964) *Sanity, Madness and the Family.* London: Tavistock.

National Institute for Clinical Excellence (2002) *Clinical Guidelines. Core Interventions in the Treatment and Management of Schizophrenia in Primary and Secondary Care.* London: NICE.

Nolan P (1993) *A History of Mental Health Nursing.* London: Chapman Hall.

Nolan P (2000) History of mental health nursing and psychiatry. In: R Newell and K Gournay (eds) *Mental Health Nursing. An Evidence-based Approach.* Edinburgh: Churchill Livingstone.

Nursing and Midwifery Council (2002) *An NMC Guide for Students of Nursing and Midwifery.* London: NMC.

Nursing and Midwifery Council (2004) *Code of Professional Conduct: Standards for Conduct, Performance and Ethics.* London: NMC.

Nursing and Midwifery Council (2005) *Students – Guidance on Clinical Experience.* London: NMC.

Onyett S (2004) Functional teams and whole systems. In: I Norman and I Ryrie (eds) *The Art and Science of Mental Health Nursing. A Textbook of Principles and Practice.* Maidenhead: Open University Press.

Porter R (2002) *Madness. A Brief History.* Oxford: Oxford University Press.

Ritter S (1997) Taking stock of psychiatric nursing. In: S Tilley (ed) *The Mental Health Nurse. Views of Practice and Education.* Oxford: Blackwell Science.

Sainsbury Centre for Mental Health (2000) *The Capable Practitioner. A Framework and List of the Practitioner Capabilities required to Implement the National Service Framework for Mental Health.* London: SCMH.

Szasz T (1961) *The Myth of Mental Illness.* New York: Dell.

UKCC (1986) *Project 2000: A New Preparation for Practice.* London: UKCC.

UKCC (1999) *Fitness for Practice. The UKCC Commission for Nursing and Midwifery Education.* London: UKCC.

www.dh.gov.uk/policyandguidance/healthandsocialcaretopics/mentalhealth

www.nelh.nhs.uk/cochrane

www.nice.org.uk

www.scmh.org.uk/80256FBD004F6342/vWeb/pcKHAL65CGBG

www.skillsforhealth.org.uk/mentalhealth

Section 1
Essential skills

2

Therapeutic relationships

If you can form a therapeutic relationship with your patient, anything else is icing on the cake.

Third year student nurse

INTRODUCTION

The therapeutic relationship is central to mental health nursing. Everything that happens between the nurse and the patient takes place within the relationship between them. It begins the moment they meet as they 'size each other up' and register their own reactions to each other, but it cannot be taken for granted as relationships of any sort require an investment of energy. Mental health patients are often characterized by relationship difficulties, and so the development of a relationship that is perceived to be therapeutic requires particular skill and attention on the part of the nurse. The more 'therapeutic' the quality of the relationship, the more likely you are to be able to work together productively for the welfare of the patient.

In this chapter, we define 'therapeutic relationship' by exploring the components of relationships in general and considering the particular 'therapeutic' aspects of the relationship. We then outline the four key issues with which therapeutic relationships are concerned: these are power and control, partnership, boundaries and core conditions. We conclude by exploring the stages of progression of a therapeutic relationship from its inception to its end.

RELATIONSHIPS

We all have experience of relationships. Throughout our lives, we come into contact with many people, but we would not claim to have 'relationships' with them all. For example, we encounter people when we buy things from them in shops or when we travel on public transport, but we would only describe our contact with them as a 'relationship' if we began to develop some sense of who they are and to share something of our own personality with them.

Usually, our relationships begin with people we are 'given', such as parents, siblings or other family members. As we grow up, we are gradually exposed to relationships with an increasing range of people. These may be with people we choose, such as our friends, or with people we encounter, such as work colleagues. Each of these relationships is unique to the people involved, but many of them are defined by the role of the other person, or by our role in relation to them. For example, a relationship with a teacher is very different from a relationship with a brother. Yet, relationships with teachers are not all the same; because our personality and that of each teacher interacts differently, we may feel friendly towards some and more fearful of others. But there is a similar quality to our relationships with all teachers, which is to do with their role as a 'teacher' and ours as 'pupils' or 'students'.

Characteristics of relationships

Relationships are 'reciprocal', that is they involve give and take. This means that both the people involved are hoping to gain something, as well as to give something. Although all relationships are unique because of the different personalities and circumstances involved, there are five key characteristics that are common to all relationships. Although some of the characteristics may seem very practical, they all have an emotional element. They can be thought of as issues with which each relationship is concerned to a greater or lesser extent.

Attachment or connection

Attachment or connection refers to the emotional connection between the participants in a relationship. Usually, we think of strong emotional connections between family members, particularly between a mother and child, which persist throughout life. For example, in most relationships with close family, there are emotional bonds between people. This is sometimes clearer during periods of separation from each other. It does not depend on closeness, fondness or even liking between people as it relates to the emotional bond we feel for what the other person represents rather than the person themselves. Some relationships, usually close family ones, are bound by very strong attachments, while others are less rigid and may change over time, for example your relationship with a fellow student may last only while you are studying together.

Commitment

Commitment relates to the level of emotional investment each participant places in the relationship. A relationship with a partner or spouse usually involves a high level of emotional investment, whereas a casual acquaintance may require little or none. Other relationships are less clearly defined in this respect. For example, a relationship with a work colleague may imply a high emotional investment, but it may be that the investment is to the 'job' rather than to the person.

Interdependence

Interdependence is the degree to which each participant is dependent on the other. This may be both emotional and financial dependency. For example, children are usually emotionally and financially dependent on their parents, whereas business partners may be less aware of an emotional dependency, but acutely conscious of their financial ones. Interdependency implies a 'give and take' within the relationship, where the participants may have different needs that they rely on the other person to meet. For example, couples sometimes adopt stereotypical roles, where one is mainly responsible for maintaining the home while the other is mainly concerned with providing the income. Practical interdependency is relatively easy to identify, but emotional dependency issues are more difficult to see. For example, in health care, a patient is usually dependent on the nurse, but the nurse also relies on the patient for employment as well as emotional gains such as work satisfaction and personal feedback.

Use of resources

This is concerned with both the access we gain to the resources of the other person and the access we allow to ours. Resources may be physical, such as our home, money or car, as well as more abstract resources such as our skills and ideas. The relationship is characterized by the extent to which these resources are shared within the relationship. Close personal relationships may demand a sharing of resources such as home and money, as well as personal resources, whereas work relationships may call for resources such as skills and ideas. In turn, we expect to access the resources of those with whom we have relationships to a degree that reflects the level of the relationship. This is an important social indicator. If somebody makes a demand on our resources beyond the boundary of the relationship, they acknowledge this by asking a 'favour', and they are expected to demonstrate their gratitude. If they fail to do this adequately, we may feel offended or feel that they have been intrusive or overfamiliar. If someone else, with whom we have a different relationship (e.g. a son or daughter), makes the same demand, we may be surprised that they regard it as a favour at all, as it falls within our perception of the shared resource.

Change

Change is the fifth characteristic and relates to both the way that relationships change to accommodate the changes in the participants, and the way the relationship brings about changes in the participants. Meeting new people and developing relationships with them can change our outlook on things and change the way we see ourselves and the world. Equally, changes in us and our circumstances alter the balance in our relationships, and this needs to be accommodated. For example, if your best friend meets someone and falls in love, this will have an effect on your friendship (Box 2.1).

Activity box 2.1 Characteristics of relationships

Think about the relationships in your life, e.g. with family, friends and other students. How are their characteristics similar to or different from each other?

THERAPEUTIC RELATIONSHIPS

What distinguishes a therapeutic relationship from other sorts of relationship is its specific position between a person who needs a certain sort of help and a person who can provide it, in this case a patient and a nurse. It simultaneously implies two inter-related ideas about the nature of the relationship. First, that the helper, or nurse, attends to the needy person, or patient. In this sense, nurses, and particularly mental health nurses working in asylums, were once known as attendants. To attend to something suggests giving it care, thought and attention. This includes both attending to the patient's physical needs (e.g. nutrition or personal hygiene) and paying attention to them in the sense of listening.

The second idea relates to the way someone is treated, that is how the other person behaves towards them. Nurses are not at liberty to behave as they wish but must act or treat patients in accordance with their professional code. The way that you treat a person is similar to the idea of attending to them. However, it also implies treatment that is provided to relieve or cure some disease, with healing or curative properties, such as a particular medication. A relationship that is therapeutic encompasses both these ideas. It is both attentive to the concerns of the patient and includes particular ideas about how the patient is to be treated, that is with equality, empathy, dignity and respect.

From this, it is clear that the relationship is the key tool at the nurse's disposal, and through it the work of nursing takes place. However, this also suggests that the relationship itself plays a healing role, indicating that the relationship is central and the 'therapy', or what the nurse does, is secondary. This may seem surprising, but research has consistently shown that the most important factor in the therapeutic relationship is the patients' perception of the quality of the relationship. If the patient feels that the relationship is a good one (therapeutic), then there is a better chance of success (Roth & Fonagy 2005).

The patient's perception of the quality of the nurse–patient relationship is based largely on how the nurse communicates. Some of this communication takes place verbally, in speech, and some in body language, but behaviour is also an important part. For example, a nurse who consistently turns up late or cancels meetings may be communicating that the relationship is not very important. So the way the nurse behaves towards the patient, or 'treats' them, is an important ingredient of the therapeutic relationship (see Chapter 6).

PRINCIPLES OF THERAPEUTIC RELATIONSHIPS

A therapeutic relationship does not happen automatically. Many people with mental health problems experience difficulty in developing and maintaining all kinds of relationships. A therapeutic relationship is a particular kind of relationship that requires an investment of energy, attention and skill on the part of the nurse. It is a central part of the mental health nurse's role as it provides the foundation for the success of other interventions. The therapeutic relationship is not in itself an activity, as it is not focused on what the nurse does, but it is an interpersonal quality that focuses more on the way in which the nurse behaves with the patient. This encompasses aspects of the nurse's role in relation to the patient. Clearly, the relationship is very different from one of family member, but it also differs from other professional roles, such as psychiatrist or social worker. This interpersonal quality is characterized by the attitudes and values that the nurse adopts towards the patient, and the way and extent to which they communicate these.

Attitudes and values

There are four interconnected attitudes and values that affect the development of a therapeutic relationship. These are power and control, partnership, boundaries and core conditions. Before reading the next section, read the scenario in Box 2.2 and consider how issues of power and control might impact on the relationship between the patient (Carol) and the nurse (Brian).

Power and control

There are always questions of power and control to be considered between mental health nurses and their patients. Sometimes, this may be very clear, for example a patient may be detained against their will or be receiving treat-

Activity box 2.2 Issues of power and control

Carol is 22 years old. She was admitted to the acute ward 2 weeks ago, after becoming increasingly unhappy and tearful to the point where she was unable to take care of herself.

Over the last week, she has slowly begun to interact with Brian, her named nurse, and has disclosed that she does not wish to continue living as she feels she is a burden and unworthy of the attention she is receiving. She is preoccupied with her feelings of guilt and unworthiness and is constantly watchful for opportunities to harm herself.

Brian arranges for a regimen of constant supervision to be put in place to ensure that Carol is constantly accompanied by a nurse.

Consider how issues of power and control might impact on the relationship between Carol and Brian.

ment without their consent under the Mental Health Act (1983). In these circumstances, the nurse has a role as a representative of the authority restricting the patient's freedom. Some patients may feel grateful for this restriction, perceiving it to be protective, but many others may feel angry and resentful about it and blame the nurse. In either case, there is a statutory authority invested in nurses, which gives them a certain amount of control over the activities and choices that the patient can make.

At other times, the power and control issues may be more subtle. For example, the patient may be suffering from a mental health problem that affects their self-esteem, leaving them feeling vulnerable, worthless and possibly a risk to their own safety. Equally, their capacity for self-control may be impaired, leaving them at risk of acting out their aggressive or sexual impulses towards other people. In these circumstances, the patient's judgment, or their ability to take responsibility for their own safety or behaviour, is impaired, making it necessary for the nurse to step in and take control in order to maintain the safety and well-being of the patient or others.

However the power and control issues manifest themselves, they are always present and are almost always weighted in favour of the nurse. They will always have some effect on the nurse–patient relationship, although individual patients and nurses will respond to them differently.

In the scenario in Box 2.2, it is important that Brian discusses the regimen of constant supervision with Carol, explaining that the intention is to respond to her feelings that she is a danger to herself by taking the responsibility for keeping her safe until she feels able to be responsible for herself again.

Power and the nurse

It is important for nurses to be conscious of the power and control issues and to notice their own reactions to these. Any authority invested in the nurse is a temporary phenomenon, the focus of which is the welfare of the patient and restoring them to health when they can take charge of themselves again. Some nurses may find that an authoritative position feels very uncomfortable, while for others it may be more comfortable than other positions. Either way, the management of authority is an essential part of the nurse's role as it may establish important limits to the patient's behaviour, which can prevent the most distressing extremes and may sometimes be life saving. Therefore, it is important that nurses are aware of their own eagerness or reluctance in relation to the power issues so that they manage them appropriately. This is an issue that can usefully be explored in clinical supervision (see Chapter 5).

Power and the patient

It is also important for the nurse to have an understanding of the patient's reaction to the power and control issues because they affect the relationship and will play a role in its therapeutic effects. For example, although a patient may appear to be co-operating with their care, they may actually be resentful of what they perceive to be intrusion by the service which the nurse represents. This is important because patients will not be committed to the work they are undertaking, and this will undermine its effectiveness. Resentment may be even more apparent when a patient is being treated against their will. At the other extreme, patients may be complying with the perceived authority of the nurse and therefore not actively participating in the relationship. In order for the work to be effective, the patient needs to feel an investment in it but, if they are simply 'going along with' the care plan because they feel unable to question it or disagree, their commitment will be weak.

Partnership

Working in partnership with patients, service users and their families is a key principle of modern mental health care (Department of Health 2004). The first step is to engage with patients or service users and carers, and the most effective way to do this is to focus on issues that are important to them. When the nurse and patient are in agreement about what is important, engagement is relatively straightforward. At times, the nurse and the patient will hold quite different views, and managing this becomes much more challenging for the nurse. As discussed above, if there are concerns about the patient's safety, these must take priority. Sometimes, the relationship may take a long time to develop even though the nurse is offering time and paying attention to what the patient wants. The nurse needs to be patient and manage the frustration they may feel about how long it is taking, and realize that this is a vital part of developing a relationship in which it is possible to work together.

Partnership concerns the degree to which patients are involved in their own care. There are two aspects to this issue: the way that nurses facilitate or provide opportunities for the patient to be involved; and the extent to which a patient puts themselves forward to be involved. However, this is not as straightforward as it might seem as both the patient and the nurse are subject to pressures that make partnership working challenging.

Partnership means there are two issues to consider. The first is the patient's right to self-determination. As long as we do not harm others, all of us, including patients, have the right to live our lives according to our own priorities and choices. The second is that the care is more likely to have a successful outcome if the patient is committed to it, and this, in turn, is more likely if it addresses issues of real concern to the patient in ways that they understand.

The promotion of partnership working requires a deliberate facilitative process on the part of the nurse. Partnership is concerned with accommodating the patient's view into the assessment and requires the nurse to take a genuine interest in the patient's thoughts and ideas. This requires the nurse to listen and attend closely to the patient's wishes and to share the decision-making responsibility. This should result in care planning that is adapted to the patient. Partnership is not concerned with persuading or manipulating the patient to accept the nurse's assessment.

Challenges to partnership working

There are organizational and safety concerns that may make partnership working challenging for nurses. Part of the nurse's role is to assess and maintain the patients' safety, and this may mean that the patient is subject to restrictions either imposed or administered by the nurse.

Restrictions and supervision

Some patients will need to be continuously supervised, with a nurse in close proximity throughout the day and night, or a patient's freedom may be restricted within prescribed parameters, such as an allowance of a 15-minute 'pass' to visit to a shop. These can be very unpleasant and intrusive experiences for patients, which few would be likely to choose freely.

These restrictions place the nurse in a position of power and authority where it is difficult to incorporate the patient's perspective, and patients may legitimately ask questions about the purpose and necessity of these restrictions. It is vital that the nurse considers whether such measures address concerns that are real to the patient and whether they are the best way of addressing these concerns. If the patient understands that the invasion of their privacy that is inherent in continuous supervision is a countermeasure to their sudden or ongoing suicidal impulses, they may be more able to perceive the intervention as useful and protective. Furthermore, the patient may bring an alternative view to situations and may have fresh ideas about how these issues could be addressed, which might otherwise not occur to the nurse. These ideas should be given real consideration and, if possible, incorporated into the care plan, but it must always be remembered that the patient's safety cannot be compromised.

Patient non-participation

Patients may find it difficult to participate fully in their care, and it is important for the nurse to be sensitive to this. The reasons for non-participation fall into three main categories: symptoms, disempowerment and disagreement. It is important to try to distinguish between the reasons for non-participation as they may require subtly different responses. It is particularly important not to confuse a 'disagreement' with 'symptoms' and to distinguish a 'disagreement' difficulty from one which is motivated by 'disempowerment'.

Symptoms The patient's ability to make judgements and choices may be impeded by the symptoms of their illness. This stretches along a spectrum of symptoms, from the patient who feels worthless and hopeless and has little volition to engage with the process of assessment and planning, through the patient who has a cognitive impairment and may not understand the nurse's interventions, to the patient whose understanding of the world makes it difficult for them to trust the motivations of the nurse. A thorough assessment should clarify whether and how symptoms are impacting on the patient.

Disempowerment   Nurses are invested with power simply because they are nurses; their professional status implies knowledge and expertise which non-nurses do not have. This may leave the patient feeling relatively unknowledgeable about their own health and therefore disempowered in relation to their care. Many patients do have extensive knowledge of how mental illness affects them as well as knowing what helps them to cope and recover. Nurses should seek to draw on this knowledge before offering solutions or giving advice.

Disagreement   Patients may perceive their situation and difficulties differently from the nurse. They may simply not agree with the nurse's assessment, or they may conceptualize the issues differently, emphasizing other factors and espousing different interventions that might seem unrealistic, pointless or irrelevant to the nurse. This disagreement may be based on a real difference in perception between the nurse and the patient, or it may be an expression of the patient's feeling of disempowerment.

Boundaries

Relationships of all sorts are defined within a set of 'boundaries' (see also Chapter 4). They describe what kind of relationship it is and provide the rules and expectations that govern it. For example, two people who work in the same place may get to know each other. In talking about their relationship, they may call themselves 'work colleagues', which has different connotations from calling themselves 'friends who work together'. We understand that we are likely to have different expectations of our friends compared with the people with whom we work, and we understand that there are limits to what we can expect of work colleagues. This applies to all relationships.

Boundaries establish the definition of the relationship: what it is for and what its rules are. In most relationships, we take these for granted and rarely discuss the boundary issues, but there are times when we become more aware of them. For example, when people are attracted to each other, it is sometimes unclear at what point they stop being 'friends' and start being 'a couple'. Equally, in friendship, we can sometimes be surprised or bewildered to find that others have a different understanding of the definition of the relationship, or of its rules. For example, if we find that something told in confidence has been disclosed to a third party, we feel betrayed and wonder how we could have trusted that person with our confidence.

The same principle applies in a therapeutic relationship. The boundaries define what the relationship is and what it is not. A therapeutic relationship is focused on the health and welfare of the patient. It is not a friendship or any other social relationship. It exists because of the patient's needs, specifically to help to address those needs. Such clarity about the definition of the relationship helps to clarify what behaviours and expectations are acceptable and appropriate to it, and what belongs elsewhere.

It is important that both the nurse and the patient understand the nature of the relationship, but it is not unusual to find that there is confusion among both nurses and patients about this. A patient might ask a direct question about a nurse's private life, and the nurse may be unsure about how to respond. This illustrates a lack of clarity about what is appropriate in the relationship and what is not and may reflect a deeper misunderstanding about what the relationship is for. They may be confused about where the boundary between a therapeutic relationship and friendship falls. The boundaries define this and stop the relationship merging into friendship or sexual intimacy and keep the focus on the therapeutic work.

In the scenario outlined in Box 2.3, the nurse should be clear that it is not possible to meet the patient following discharge as this would imply a shift from a professional relationship to a personal one. The nurse could thank the patient for the invitation but say that it is not possible to meet them once they have been discharged. This type of situation is complex and needs to be handled sensitively. It would be important to acknowledge that there had

 Activity box 2.3 Boundaries

You are working on a ward and allocated to a patient who is a similar age to you. You have spent a lot of time with this patient and are aware that you have many common interests as well as a similar view of the world and a shared sense of humour.

The patient is about to be discharged and asks you if you would like to meet for a coffee once they leave hospital.

Think about how you would respond to this.

been a sharing of interests and values that can bring a sense of closeness and connection. It is possible that the request might reveal a need for new friendships that could form part of the therapeutic work between the nurse and the patient. The nurse should also reflect on whether there was anything they might have said or done that might have made the boundaries of the relationship seem unclear.

Core conditions of a therapeutic relationship

American psychologist Carl Rogers (1951) suggested that a therapeutic relationship has three essential ingredients and that the more these ingredients are present, the more therapeutic the relationship. Rogers (1957) later wrote that these ingredients were 'necessary and sufficient', that is they are essential to the relationship and nothing more is needed. Others (e.g. Egan 2002) believe that other knowledge and skills are also needed, but most agree that Rogers' three ingredients are necessary (if not sufficient), and they have become known as the 'core conditions' of a therapeutic relationship.

The core conditions are 'attitudes' which the nurse (or therapist) adopts and expresses in their dealings with the patient. They are empathy, genuineness and acceptance. It is sometimes difficult to maintain these attitudes, and they are not absolute. The idea is to adopt them as much as you can and to express them to the patient.

Empathy

Empathy means the attempt to understand the other person in a deep way. To try and set aside one's own judgements and preconceptions and to understand how the other person experiences things. To gain an understanding of their thoughts and feelings and what these mean to them. A key part of the presence of empathy in the relationship is that the nurse communicates their empathic understanding to the patient. It may be difficult to understand how the patient feels about things, but it is important to try and to let the patient know that you are trying.

The simplest way of letting the patient know what you have understood is to tell them. You are not the patient and do not have the same emotions and experiences as them, so it would probably not be true to say that you understand; it may be more useful to tell the patient what you have understood, to reflect back or to summarize what they have said. This may be what you have understood from what has been said, or it may be what you have inferred from their behaviour. You do not necessarily have to get it exactly right, or to have a perfect summary of the patient's feelings. What you need to do is to let the patient know that you are trying to understand them. If you are not quite right, the patient will usually correct you or clarify their feelings.

Genuineness

Genuineness refers to the extent to which the nurse is able to be honest in the relationship in a 'real' way. Nurses need to have an awareness of their own thoughts and feelings when they are with the patient, and to engage in the relationship as a real person with these thoughts and feelings. This does not mean necessarily telling the patient how you feel, but it does mean noticing how you feel and accepting it. This can be confusing for nurses because of boundaries and roles, but it is not about developing a personal relationship or acting a part. For example, if you are aware of having a feeling of dislike towards a patient, you would not be expected to act this out towards the patient, but it may be that there is something about how they relate to people which engenders this reaction. It may be useful for the patient to know about this at some point, but it would probably not be helpful just to tell them outright. Neither would it be helpful to encourage them to feel that you were very fond of them.

Genuineness requires the nurse to 'wear' their role rather like a uniform, which maintains the formal nature of the relationship. Genuineness means that nurses remain themselves, aware of their own reactions and feelings, while also being a nurse (see 'Boundaries' p. 35 and Chapter 4). Genuineness calls for the nurse to be tactful but honest in their relations with the patient as this is the foundation of a trusting relationship.

Acceptance

Acceptance is the positive respect a nurse has for their patient. It means that nurses accept that people simply are who they are and have a right to be respected for it. It also assumes that people are not wilfully bad or unpleasant, but are doing their best to manage in their particular circumstances.

This idea can be challenging for mental health nurses who may, for example, be working in a forensic setting with patients who have committed crimes that the nurse finds abhorrent. The point is not that the nurse is wrong or should not have that feeling or should forget about the crime but, rather, that the nurse's personal judgement is not helpful to the patient. Telling a smoker that we dislike and disapprove of smoking does not help him to stop, but accepting that he does smoke and exploring with him his motivation and feelings about it may help him to feel differently about it. Similarly, telling a patient who has committed a serious sexual assault that he shouldn't have done it is unlikely to be helpful, whereas exploring with him how and why it came about may be.

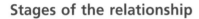

Stages of the relationship

Therapeutic relationships are temporary phenomena associated with periods in the patient's life when they need particular kinds of help and support, which can be provided by nurses. By definition, at the outset of their relationship, the patient will have needs that they no longer have when the relationship ends. This may not mean that all the patient's needs have been met; it may mean that they are better equipped with the resources to achieve this without the nurse's help. On the other hand, it may simply mean that the patient's needs have changed and are now of a type that *this* nurse can no longer help with, but a nurse in a different role (or other professional) may be better placed to help with the new needs (for example, a patient discharged from an acute ward to the care of a community mental health nurse).

Peplau (1952) suggested that between meeting and parting, the relationship passes through four different phases as the patient progresses towards recovery: orientation; identification; exploitation and resolution. Although each phase can be described separately from the others, in practice they are not distinct, but merge into one another. Nor is there a timeframe for progressing from one phase to another; in fact, Simpson (1991) suggests that each phase has defined tasks and that some of the earlier phases may be repeated if the patient's needs change.

Orientation

In the orientation phase, the patient makes adjustments, or gets used to, their new situation. They have to adjust to the condition of their health, new people and relationships, and possibly new surroundings and restrictions on their liberty. These are all significant adjustments which may take time to achieve.

A person who develops a mental health problem will have their own understanding of the experience. Someone who has previous experience may understand that they are beginning to relapse and that they need to seek help, while others may be reluctant to do so for fear of the consequences. Another group may simply be unaware that their experiences can be described as the symptoms of a mental health problem, either because it has never happened to them before or because it doesn't occur to them that they may be relapsing. Once their problem has been recognized and they are beginning to receive care, they need to get used to the new circumstances.

The first phase of the therapeutic relationship helps the patient to adjust to the new understanding of what has happened to them, and to come to terms with their feelings about this. Some may be relieved that their condition can be recognized and treated, while others may be disappointed that they have not been able to stay well. Still others may be angry at what they perceive as an unwarranted intrusion into their life. The nurse helps to facilitate this process by being available to help explore the patient's reactions and to provide information when appropriate.

The patient may also be faced with a bewildering set of new people; the nurse is one, but there may also be other professionals involved. If the patient has been admitted to hospital, there will also be other patients to contend with. It takes time to develop trust and confidence in people, even doctors and nurses, particularly if you feel quite miserable and would rather be left alone, or if you are fearful that someone may be trying to harm you. The patient needs to adjust to these relationships, and the nurse can facilitate this by listening and becoming a familiar and supportive companion.

Linked to the difficulty of adjusting to new people is the need to adjust to new surroundings. If a patient has been admitted to hospital, or transferred from one setting to another, they will take a little time to get used to it. They may be alarmed by the idea of being in a mental hospital, and all the stereotypical ideas they have about this. They also need to learn the geography, the routine and the rules, and the nurse can help by being understanding about their disorientation and reminding them about things if they need it.

In this phase, the nurse is primarily concerned with maintaining the patient's safety and with presenting themselves to the patient as trustworthy and supportive.

Identification

Once patients have begun to adjust to their new circumstances, they can begin to develop a better understanding of their problems and needs. The identification phase is where the partnership (see p. 32) aspect of the relationship comes into play, as the patient and nurse begin to work together to identify how the patient is affected by their mental health problem and what help and support they need from the nurse. The nurse and patient collaborate to assess comprehensively the way in which the patient has been affected by their mental health problem and to work out ways in which the nurse can be helpful. From this assessment, they negotiate a care plan.

Exploitation

The exploitation phase is the working phase of the relationship. This is where the patient takes advantage of (exploits) their understanding gained in the orientation and identification phases, the structure provided by the nurse–patient relationship and the negotiated care plan to manage or overcome the difficulties imposed by their mental health problems in collaboration with the nurse. This does not happen suddenly; the patient may have difficult or longstanding problems that require a significant change in outlook or behaviour and may need a number of stages centred around a sequence of short-term goals leading towards the overall target.

The exploitation phase is dynamic as the original assessment and care plans are regularly revisited and renegotiated in response to the patient's changing health. The nurse needs to be sensitive to the patient's changing level of dependency and to respond by moving towards facilitating the patient, rather than intervening on their behalf, as they become less dependent.

Resolution

The resolution phase is where the patient has achieved a level of health where they no longer require the support of this nurse. Their original nursing problems are resolved and they are moving on, either to another therapeutic relationship with another nurse in a different role or to care for themselves independently. It is the ending phase of the relationship where the patient develops a renewed sense of their own independence and is able to appreciate the care they have received, but realize they no longer need it. This can be difficult for nurses as they also need to recognize and accept the patient's renewed competency.

SUMMARY

- Relationships are characterized by attachment, commitment, interdependence, use of resources and change.
- A therapeutic relationship is a temporary phenomenon that is concerned with, and attentive to, the welfare of the patient.
- The patient's perception of the quality of the relationship is based on how the nurse communicates.
- In a therapeutic relationship, the nurse has to manage the power imbalance between nurse and patient and set the boundaries of the relationship.
- Boundaries establish the definition of the relationship, what it's for and what its rules are.
- Empathy, genuineness and acceptance are the core conditions of a therapeutic relationship.
- A therapeutic relationship progresses through four phases: orientation, identification, exploitation and resolution.

References

Department of Health (2004) *The Ten Essential Shared Capabilities. A Framework for the Whole of the Mental Health Workforce*. London: Department of Health.

Egan G (2002) *The Skilled Helper: A Problem Management and Opportunity Development Approach to Helping*, 7th edn. Pacific Grove, CA: Brooks/Cole Publishing.

Peplau H (1952) *Interpersonal Relations in Nursing*. New York: GP Putnam.

Rogers C (1951) *Client Centered Therapy*. London: Constable.

Rogers C (1957) *On Becoming a Person: A Therapist's View of Psychotherapy*. London: Constable.

Roth A, Fonagy P (2005) *What Works for Whom?*, 2nd edn. New York: Guilford Publications.

Simpson H (1991) *Peplau's Model in Action*. London: Macmillan.

3

Observation

> *It's amazing what you notice when you start to pay attention. I've started to notice more about myself as well as the patients.*
>
> Second year student nurse

INTRODUCTION

Observation is something that we all do all the time. Whether we are meeting friends, going for a job interview or standing in a queue at a supermarket checkout or bus stop, we are constantly observing others, the environment and ourselves. If going for an interview, we are likely to notice that we are excited, anxious or frustrated and will have checked to see that we have dressed appropriately. When we meet friends, we notice whether they look well and happy or sad, and we scan the environment for signs of a traffic jam or accident that might indicate we will have to wait even longer for the bus.

In such situations, much of our observation is automatic, and we do not even think about it. Observation provides us with data that helps us to function effectively in the world, especially in our relationships with others. It is also essential for our safety; for example, if there is a fire, it is important to be able to notice the smell of smoke and the source of heat. Similarly, if we are injured, it is important to be able to notice the location and severity of the wound. In these situations, our observations provide us with information; we then have to decide how to act on this information.

Observation is such an essential skill that mental health nurses are sometimes referred to as 'trained observers'. In this chapter, we explain what we mean by observation, why it is important and how it is related to assessment. We also provide you with some principles, frameworks and guidance for observing yourself, others and the environment.

WHAT IS OBSERVATION?

In mental health nursing, observation has two linked but distinct meanings; observation means noticing or perceiving, but it is also used to describe a nursing intervention. According to dictionary definitions, the word observation refers to noticing and perception as well as accurate watching and noting of one's self, others and the environment. For nurses, the reason for observing is to collect data to plan, implement and evaluate care. This happens through the radar-like quality of our senses that collect information about the world. 'Noticing' is an active or purposeful process of attending to some aspects of the sensory information. Noticing is a general life skill, and everybody has this ability to notice or observe, although some people are more observant than others.

As nurses, we need to develop and refine these skills so that we notice the pertinent aspects of a situation. This includes noticing ourselves, the patient's appearance, behaviour and speech and the environment in which the situation occurs. Observation will take place in a variety of settings including the patient's home, wards and clinics as well as more public settings, for example a café or park.

Observation as an intervention

In mental health nursing, the word 'observation' is also used to describe an intervention that is most frequently applied in an inpatient setting. It is used in situations in which there is a risk that the patient may behave in a way that causes harm to themselves or others. In this type of observation (often referred to as close or special observation), the nurse has to ensure that the patient is within eyesight or even closer, for example within arm's length, in order to prevent harm to themselves or others. This is a highly specialized application of observation, which we discuss briefly in the section on observation of others (see p. 49). For the purposes of this book, we are using the word observation to represent a general skill rather than a specific intervention. In general nursing, the term observation is also used to mean the measurement of vital signs such as temperature, pulse and blood pressure.

How do we observe?

Unlike many aspects of mental health nursing (e.g. giving medication or making a mental health assessment), observation is something we are already able to do when we start nursing. As with all the skills and abilities that we already possess, it is important to reflect on these to assess whether they match the skills needed to be a nurse. This raises a number of questions such as: how do I make observations now? As a nurse, can I continue in the same way or will I need to change how I observe? Do the exercise in Box 3.1 (overleaf).

It is likely that your description will have included some introductory material such as the names of the characters and their relationships to each other. You may also have described aspects of their appearance such as clothing, as well as commenting on how they spoke and behaved. What else did you say? Did you comment on their motives or make judgements about whether they were a 'good' or a 'bad' character? In our personal lives, as well as making observations, we have a tendency to read into or interpret what we observe. In nursing, we also interpret information or data, but we must be wary of jumping to conclusions or drawing inferences that are based on our beliefs and not on what we have actually observed. So, think back to what you described and try to separate observation from speculation or interpretation.

Activity box 3.1 **Describing a television programme**

Get together with a friend or relative and think back to a recent episode of a favourite television programme – focus on just one scene.

Describe what you observed in this scene to the other person.

Make a few notes about what you said.

Observation is based on information drawn from our senses. We mostly use our sight and hearing to collect information about someone else's appearance, behaviour and speech. If we have some physical contact, for example by shaking hands, we may also receive information about the person's temperature. The final sense that we may use is the sense of smell. Sometimes, we may register a strong smell when we are with someone, for example we might notice that they smell strongly of body odour or aftershave or perfume. Often, what we are noticing, but may not make explicit, is that we are not noticing any particular smell through our olfactory sense. The sense of smell is one that we draw on more often when we are observing the environment. It is particularly important in helping us to manage our safety, for example in detecting smoke or gas or determining whether food is safe to eat.

THE PROCESS OF OBSERVATION

In mental health nursing, the process of observation has three components: observing, reporting and recording (Figure 3.1). Observing involves noticing oneself, the patient and others, and the environment, and this requires perceptual and interaction skills. Reporting incorporates reasoning skills and the ability to present the results of your observation, and the ability to record information may draw on presentational and summarizing skills (Ritter 1989).

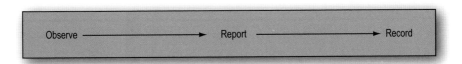

Figure 3.1 The process of observation.

Observation of self

As a mental health nurse, you need to develop the capacity to observe yourself, particularly in relation to your work with patients. Awareness of yourself, or self-observation, is important for two reasons. First, it provides you with some clues about the effect you may have on others and they on you. For example, if you are feeling bad tempered or irritable, this is likely to affect the way you approach an interaction with a patient. Similarly, if you are feeling tired and vulnerable, you may be more susceptible than usual to the effects of the behaviour of others. By being aware of this, you have the potential to modify the impact of your mood state on the patient. Secondly, your reactions to another person are a source of potentially useful and important information. Filtering out these reactions, either because you think they are not important or because you feel awkward or embarrassed about your feelings (of like or dislike, for example), means this information could be lost and result in an incomplete assessment. We explore this further in the chapter on therapeutic relationships (Chapter 2).

Observation of feelings and emotions

In relation to observing yourself, there are two aspects to notice. The first relates to the internal world represented by your thoughts and feelings. This involves paying attention to your reactions to patients as well as colleagues. Notice, for example, how you feel about them, whether you like them or not, and think about what it is you like or dislike. These feelings might be to do with your own unique reactions to a patient (for example you might feel attracted to someone), and this may affect the way you behave towards them. Other staff and patients might have similar feelings and reactions, so your response could provide important information about the patient, which should not be lost. Be aware too if you find yourself thinking about a patient outside the working environment. Although it is not uncommon to do this, especially when we are new and inexperienced, it should not reach a level where it becomes a preoccupation.

Observation of behaviour

The second area to pay attention to relates to your behaviour. Be aware of how you find yourself behaving towards patients. Notice, for example, whether you find yourself joking with them or drawn in to having intimate conversations; you might feel protective towards them or perhaps a little anxious or scared of them. Consider the relationship between your thoughts and feelings and behaviour. For example, if you like one of the patients, notice whether you seek their company or whether your feelings concern you and make you try to keep your distance. Similarly, if you find yourself feeling fearful of a patient, observe whether you approach them or if you try and avoid them.

It is important to be aware that we cannot control the thoughts and feelings we have in response to other people including patients. Although our feelings may sometimes cause us to feel uncomfortable, our feelings alone will not breach any professional code. However, it is important to remember that, as nurses, we do have a *Code of Professional Conduct* (Nursing and Midwifery Council 2004) to which we must adhere and to ensure that our speech and behaviour do not contravene this in any way. The *Guidelines for Mental Health and Learning Disabilities Nursing* (UKCC 1998) specifically address the issue of relationships and make it clear that it is the nurse's responsibility to maintain appropriate boundaries (see p. 35).

Observation of the environment

There are two reasons for observing the environment. The first is to provide information about potential hazards in order to contribute to the assessment and management of environmental risks. The second is that it is important to gain information about a patient's reaction to the level of stimulation in the environment in order to help provide an environment that is neither over- nor understimulating. The environment should be assessed in relation to physical and psychological factors.

Physical factors

In clinical environments such as wards, clinics and other care settings, physical hazards such as blocked fire exits or spillages should be easy to identify and remedy. Nurses must be aware that, at times, there may be patients who are actively seeking to harm themselves. This requires paying particular attention to risks such as window openings on upper floors, identifying possible points that may be used to secure clothing, bedding or other materials to form a tie that someone might use to hang themselves from (ligature points) and ensuring medication is taken and not being secretly hoarded.

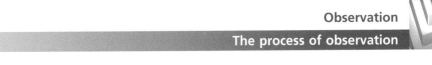

The ward environment also includes people. Nurses need to know who is on the ward at all times in order to provide a safe environment. This includes patients, staff and visitors and will be affected by the ease with which people can enter and leave. At times, it may be necessary to refuse entry to someone, for instance a visitor whom a patient does not wish to see. As a student, you can contribute to producing a safe environment by ensuring that, whenever you open the door to visitors in a clinical area, you politely ask them to identify themselves.

Psychological factors

It is important for nurses to observe and manage the environment in relation to the amount of stimulation it provides. Environments that are noisy and busy, especially at night, can be extremely unsettling. Conversely, environments may be too quiet and understimulating, and this can also have a detrimental effect on patients. The nurse must be constantly alert and vigilant and observe the environment in order to make any changes that may be necessary. Ideally, wards should have a variety of spaces available to patients including a television or music room as well as a quiet room. Having a structured programme of activities, both on and off the ward, helps to combat the boredom that patients often describe in inpatient settings.

One of the key roles of the nurse is to assist and support patients to manage the boundary between them and the environment when they are unable to manage these themselves. For example, nurses can monitor the volume of TV and sound systems, and intervene to reduce them as well as ensuring that they are only used in appropriate areas. At times, patients may need to be encouraged to leave an environment that they are finding it difficult to cope with. An example of this might be patients who believe they are receiving messages from the TV that are disturbing, or those that find someone else's behaviour is making them feel irritable or upset.

Observation of others

As a student nurse, you will work with many people including patients and service users, their family and friends and colleagues but, in this section, we are focusing specifically on how to observe patients. It is crucial for nurses to be aware of and to be able to describe what they see and hear in relation to the patient in order to gather data to plan care. Nursing observation of patients is primarily concerned with gathering data about how they are and how they interact with others and their environment. It is also about being aware of their safety, as their own ability to be aware of this may be impaired by illness, thereby placing them at risk. Unfortunately, observation is not a neutral activity; it is readily subject to bias. However, being aware of this can help to reduce some of the bias we might otherwise bring to the situation. These biases can act as 'filters' and affect how we observe. There are two specific filters we bring to observing others that can distort what we see: our culture and the way that we perceive the 'patient'.

The effect of culture

Our own cultural context gives us a sense of what fits in with or is consistent with our cultural norms. What we notice is often dictated by our cultural expectations; for instance, we may become aware of a person's eye contact if it differs from our usual social pattern but, if it is similar to our own, it may be more difficult to notice. Our cultural expectations may also lead us to wrongly interpret what we observe as we tend to see things in terms of our previous learning or experience. This can make us filter out some of what we observe. Nurses need to learn to avoid filtering out information and develop the skill of just noticing.

The notion of 'the patient'

The second 'filter' or distortion is to frame our observation around the idea of 'the patient'. If we perceive people only as 'patients', there is a risk of seeing everything in terms of illness. This can leave us with a very one-dimensional view of the person, with the result that many aspects of their lives and functioning are not acknowledged. This at odds with contemporary approaches to practice and may hamper the patient's recovery. It is essential to bear in mind that, while they may be patients in the context of our relationship with them, they have a whole life other than this, in which they are brothers or sisters, spouses or partners, colleagues or parents, etc.

Descriptive observation

Nurses need to notice and describe what they see in relation to the patient, others and the environment. Often, the first thing we notice about a person is the presence or absence of something; for example, we may not notice a person's clothing, but we would notice if a person is wearing no clothes and is wrapped only in bin-liners. The idea is to try and notice the presence or absence of things and describe them. This method is known as descriptive observation and consists of observing appearance, behaviour and speech.

Appearance

Observation of appearance involves observation of eye contact, facial expression, body and grooming and clothing (see Figure 3.2).

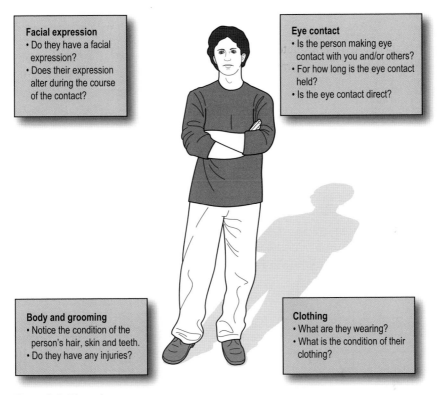

Facial expression
- Do they have a facial expression?
- Does their expression alter during the course of the contact?

Eye contact
- Is the person making eye contact with you and/or others?
- For how long is the eye contact held?
- Is the eye contact direct?

Body and grooming
- Notice the condition of the person's hair, skin and teeth.
- Do they have any injuries?

Clothing
- What are they wearing?
- What is the condition of their clothing?

Figure 3.2 Observing appearance.

Behaviour

Like appearance, behaviour is one of the key aspects of the individual that is easily observable and can provide important information about how a person is functioning. Aspects to observe are posture, movement, activity and interaction with others. At this stage, it is important just to observe without trying to interpret the behaviour.

Posture
- How do they stand, sit or lie when on their own? and with others?

Movement
- Are they moving or still?
- What is the movement and what part of the body is involved (e.g. head, trunk or limbs)?

35155

Activity
- What are they doing?
- Are they able to complete the activity (e.g. making a cup of tea)?
- Are they able to co-operate with others?

Interaction with others
- Is the person alone or with others?
- Do they listen to the people they are with and respond to their speech?
- Do they take turns in speaking?

Speech

Along with behaviour, speech is one of the main means we have to convey information about our inner world, especially the mood we are in. Observation here needs to consider the process of speech (the speed, spontaneity and volume) and the content (see Figure 3.3).

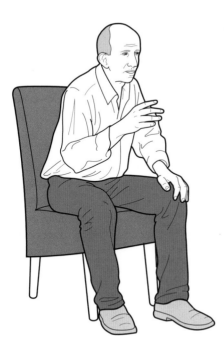

Speed and flow
- How quickly or slowly do they speak?
- Does their speech flow smoothly?
- If not, in what way?

Spontaneity and amount
- Are they speaking at all?
- Do they initiate conversation or only respond?
- How prompt are their responses?
- How much do they say?

Volume
- Can they easily be heard?
- How loudly are they speaking, are they shouting or whispering?

Content
- What are they talking about?
- Can you follow it? If not, why not?
- Is it relevant to the context (e.g. the conversation or interview situation)?

Figure 3.3 Observation of speech.

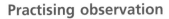

Practising observation

In order to become proficient at observation, you will need to practise the skills. Fortunately, this is relatively easy, as you do not need to be in a clinical environment to do this. As with any skill, you will find it easier to learn (and later to teach others) if it is broken down into smaller components. You could begin by looking around the room you are in and trying to describe it as factually as possible. You might watch the TV and describe what you notice about the people in an advert (most adverts are short and this can provide a good time limit). In observing others in a real-life situation, you can do this as you wait in the queue at the supermarket, noticing other shoppers or how the checkout assistant deals with the shoppers. You could start with focusing just on appearance, or even just on noticing the eye contact that people make. As your ability and confidence increase, you will be able to notice more and more and become aware of features that you might have missed at first (see Box 3.2).

Observation and interaction

Although as a student you will legitimately have the role of observer, in most mental health nursing practice, observation does not usually take place as a

---

 Activity box 3.2 Practising observation of yourself and others

Identify a situation in which you are in the role of an observer, for example a ward round, care planning approach (CPA) meeting or observing your mentor.

Decide whether to focus on observing yourself or others.

If you are **observing yourself**, see what you notice about your thoughts, feelings and behaviour in relation to what is happening.

If you are **observing others**, you can use the framework of appearance, behaviour and speech both to structure your observation and later as a checklist to see if you missed anything.

'stand alone' activity. Observation normally occurs within the context of an interaction between the nurse and the patient; otherwise, it risks being experienced as an intrusion or a form of surveillance. Nurses have to incorporate the skills of observing themselves, others and the environment at the same time as interacting with the other person.

In some settings, such as in hospital where nurses and patients are together continuously, the nurse has the opportunity for a lot of different contact with the patient. This might include formal contact in relation to assessment and treatment (for example being in a group or administering medication) as well as informal contact such as watching TV, playing games together and escorting patients outside the ward to the shops. You can use any of these situations to hone your observation skills (see Box 3.3).

REPORTING OBSERVATIONS

The next step in the process is to be able to report your observations accurately. This involves skills in verbal reporting and description as well as assessment and evaluation of risk.

Verbal reporting

Verbal reporting is the process that precedes the written recording of observations. Your observations should be reported to the person who is responsible for the care of the patient. This may be your mentor or the patient's primary nurse or key worker or, in their absence, the senior nurse on duty. The aim of the reporting process is to pass on information to a more experienced colleague who will be able to help you to 'sift' the information and decide what is important to record. They will also be able to identify any urgent pieces of information that require an immediate response.

It is important to be factual and avoid making assumptions, as these may be incorrect. Your observations may represent an incomplete picture of the patient, or you may have insufficient experience to interpret the information correctly. You should describe what you have seen and heard rather than try to explain it. Report what you have observed descriptively using ordinary language to describe your observations. Avoid using jargon, and be precise and specific but avoid being evaluative, i.e. making assumptions (see Box 3.4, p. 56).

Evaluating risk

The next step is to determine whether any of the information requires an immediate or urgent response. Anything that you consider may involve a risk

Activity box 3.3 **Observation and interaction**

When on a practice placement, choose a situation in which you plan to interact with a patient, for example discussing a TV programme you have both watched.

What do you notice about yourself as you initiate the interaction?

What do you notice about the patient (using the framework of appearance, behaviour and speech) as you approach them and begin to have contact?

What do you notice about yourself and the patient during the interaction?

Finally, be aware of your thoughts and feelings as the interaction finishes.

to the patient or others, or which you think may jeopardize the safety of the patient or others, will need to be reported immediately. If you are unsure what to do, tell someone. It is not uncommon for people to describe having a 'feeling' about something (this is also called intuition or apprehensive knowledge). This sort of information cannot always be substantiated by hard facts but is increasingly recognized as being an important type of information (Gantt & Agazarian 2005). In relation to risk, it is essential to respond to this type of information and report it to a more experienced colleague.

> **Box 3.4 An example of descriptive and evaluative reporting of behaviour and speech**
>
> *Descriptive reporting*
> Alice moved quickly back and forth across the room, picking up magazines and putting them down again without looking at them. She was talking very quickly, with frequent changes of topic in a way that was difficult to follow. Sometimes, Alice spoke in verse and occasionally broke into song. She said that she was a member of the royal family and she could hear the voice of the Queen giving her instructions to rid the world of evil.
>
> *Evaluative reporting*
> Alice was deluded and hallucinating. She was also hyperactive and overtalkative with pressure of speech and thought disorder.

Practising verbal reporting

If you can enlist some help from a friend or colleague, you can also practise your verbal reporting skills. You could start by using non-clinical material such as watching a TV advert as suggested earlier. Ask the other person to give you feedback on your reporting. In a clinical context, you could identify this in your learning contract as a skill you would like to develop and ask your mentor to give you feedback. Gradually, as you practise the skill of observation, you will start to notice yourself when you move from being descriptive to being evaluative.

RECORDING YOUR OBSERVATIONS

The final part of the process of observation is recording (documenting) in the patient's file the relevant information gleaned from your observations. You will probably not be able to write down everything that you have observed. The process of reporting your observations to a more experienced colleague may help you decide what needs to be recorded. You will also need to think about the purpose of documenting your observations and what are the relevant principles. The Nursing and Midwifery Council's (NMC) *Guidelines for Records and Record Keeping* (2005) provide a comprehensive summary of the rationale for record keeping as well as commenting on content and style, audit, legal aspects, access to records and information technology. Nurses are advised to consult this document, which is available on the NMC website at www.nmc-uk.org\aFrameDisplay.aspx?DocumentID=S16. The NMC emphasize that 'record keeping is an integral part of nursing' (NMC 2005: 5), which means that it is part of the care process and not a separate activity.

There are two main reasons for recording your observations. The first is to produce a formal record of care. The second is to provide information that contributes to the planning of future care and treatment by nurses and other professionals working in the multidisciplinary team. It is also important to consider the role of the patient or service user in relation to record keeping. As a result of legislation, most patients have rights of access to their health records. In addition, it is increasingly being recognized that their view or perspective on events should also be included as part of the record keeping process.

Principles of record keeping

There is no nationally adopted framework for record keeping, and there will be variation between health and social care organizations regarding how records are maintained. There is a move towards keeping one set of notes to which all professionals contribute, rather than having each discipline keeping their own notes that are not always readily available to others. Nonetheless, there are certain principles relating to record keeping that must be upheld (NMC 2005). This includes keeping records that are:

- factual, consistent and accurate
- written as soon as possible after an event has occurred
- written clearly and in such a manner that the text cannot be erased (i.e. written in ink)
- written in such a manner that any alterations or additions are dated, timed and signed in such a way that the original entry can still be read clearly – this means that mistakes should be crossed out with a single line so that it is clearly crossed out but still readable (correction fluid should not be used)
- accurately dated, timed and signed, with the signature printed alongside the first entry
- free of abbreviations, jargon, meaningless phrases, irrelevant speculation and offensive subjective statements
- readable on any photocopies.

OBSERVATION AND THE ESSENTIAL SKILLS

Observation is closely linked with the other essential skills of the therapeutic relationship, being able to take on different roles and reflection. Observation of self and others will mostly take place in the context of a relationship between yourself and the patient or service user. In this respect, what you observe is not just a piece of information to be taken and reported to another member of staff; you will also need to consider how to manage the observation or information in relation to the other person. One way to approach this is to think about whether you and the other person are both aware of what you have observed. For example, some information will be given to you directly by the patient through their speech and what they choose to tell you. Some information will be known to both of you, for example that they avoid making eye contact with people.

There will be additional information that you will observe but they are not aware of. For instance, someone's facial expression may suggest they feel tense or troubled but, to them, it is their usual expression and does not reflect the state that others may see.

So another part of the process of observation will be making decisions about what you have observed in relation to what should be discussed with or given as feedback to the patient. In our everyday lives, we do not react to or act upon every piece of information we come across, and the same is true when we are working with patients and service users. In the chapter on taking on different roles (Chapter 4), we discuss the importance of context and goals. For example, in the context of a first meeting, you would have to discriminate between the different information you have observed. If one of your goals is to facilitate effective communication, it would be appropriate to feed back that the other person was speaking so quietly that you could hardly hear them. We explore this more in Chapter 4.

In writing about observation, we have tried to simplify the process. However, in real life, you will have to manage a situation that is far more complex. For example, this could involve observing a patient while having a conversation, perhaps while engaged in an activity, and noticing your own reactions at the same time. Then you will have to recall what happened in order to report it to someone else. It will help your development if you are realistic about what you are likely to achieve and do not expect to be able to notice everything straight away.

SUMMARY

- Observation is a core skill for mental health nurses. The process of observation includes observing (self, others and the environment), reporting and recording.
- It is important to make observations that are based on data drawn from the senses, especially our sight and hearing.

- Observation of others involves noticing their appearance, behaviour and speech.
- Although it appears to be fairly straightforward, it is extremely difficult to notice or observe in a way that does not reflect some degree of personal or cultural bias.
- Fortunately, observation is a skill that can be readily practised. Whenever you are with people, you can 'switch on' your observer role by seeing what you notice about the people and the environment.
- Observation needs to be considered in relation to the other core skills of therapeutic relationships, taking on different roles and reflection.
- It will be necessary to interpret or make some sense of the information you have gathered, and this requires professional knowledge. There are a number of ways of doing this, which we describe in Chapter 7 on assessment.

References

Gantt SP, Agazarian YM (2005) Overview of the theory of living human systems and its systems-centered practice. In: SP Gantt and YM Agazarian (eds) *SCT in Action. Applying the Systems-Centered Approach in Organizations.* New York: iUniverse.

Nursing and Midwifery Council (2004) *Code of Professional Conduct: Standards for Conduct, Performance and Ethics.* London: NMC.

Nursing and Midwifery Council (2005) *Guidelines for Records and Record Keeping.* London: NMC.

Ritter S (1989) *Manual of Clinical Psychiatric Nursing Principles and Procedures.* London: Harper and Row.

UKCC (1998) *Guidelines for Mental Health and Learning Disabilities Nursing.* London: UKCC.

www.nmc-uk.org

4

Taking on different roles

> I've started to think that when I come to work I
> change into being a nurse but without the uniform.
> I'm still 'me' but a large part of being a nurse is
> already set out.
>
> Newly qualified staff nurse

INTRODUCTION

Becoming a mental health nurse is a new and exciting venture. It begins by taking on the role of student nurse. In some respects, it is similar to an actor taking on a part; a role helps us to identify both what something is and what it is not. Taking up different roles is part of the human experience. Within our family, we may have many roles including being a child, a sibling or a cousin. These family roles are characterized by the kinship relationship between one person and another. As we move into adulthood, we elect to take on particular roles such as parent, partner or spouse.

When we come into nursing, we bring experience, skills and abilities from our personal lives into our professional role. In some ways, the training is about helping us to identify which of our personal resources are pertinent to the role of nurse as well as developing new knowledge and skills.

In this chapter, we begin by asking you to think about the skills and abilities that you already have and can bring to nursing. We will then look at how you can effectively take up your role as a student in mental health nursing. This involves being aware of the different contexts in which the work is taking place and identifying relevant goals. Finally, we identify three core roles for mental health nurses: delivering and managing evidence-based care and interventions, providing information and managing emotions.

DEFINITION

A role relates to one's function or what one is expected to do. The word 'boundary' is commonly used in relation to roles and professional relationships (see Chapter 2, p. 35). A boundary has two important aspects. First, it incorporates the idea that something can be inside or outside the boundary. A football or other sports pitch may provide a useful analogy; here, the boundary is physically marked out. If a ball outside the touchline is kicked into the football net, it would not be counted as a goal. In nursing, the boundaries relate to defining behaviours that are acceptable or unacceptable in relation to the role. For example, shouting or swearing at a patient is not acceptable behaviour for the nurse.

The second aspect of a boundary is that is has some degree of permeability. It is essential to the survival and development of an individual or a system that it has boundaries that are sufficiently open to allow new information to be taken in. For nurses, this means that, although some aspects of the role may be quite fixed, there is also the capacity for change. This must happen at the individual level as the nurse constantly evaluates his or her practice and incorporates new learning. Similarly, the profession as a whole at the level of the Nursing and Midwifery Council (NMC) must also be receptive to change.

Some roles, or perhaps more accurately, titles, are defined in law; these include the title of nurse. In the UK, this means that no one can call themselves a Registered Nurse unless their name has been entered on the register of nurses currently held by the Nursing and Midwifery Council (www.nmc-uk.org).

Roles can be formal or informal. The expression 'a student of life' denotes someone who makes a habit of acquiring information and may take on the role of student in an informal capacity. In contrast, enrolling for a course of study involves being formally designated as a student or learner and will encompass specific expectations from an external source regarding how the student should take up the role. A formal role can only exist or operate in the context of the relationship between one person and another. For example, being a spouse or partner requires having a husband, a wife or a man or woman to whom one is also the partner. Similarly, a nurse is only able to take up the role of nurse in relation to another person such as a patient or service user, carer or other professional.

PERSONAL ROLES

In your personal life, you will already have a number of roles. Some of these will derive from your family of origin, such as child, brother or aunt. These are largely roles that are assigned to us rather than chosen, but we can decide *how* we take up the role. For example, being an aunt might involve acknowledging your niece or nephew's birthday and other significant events and attending family gatherings such as weddings and funerals, or you might choose not to do so. Cultural and social factors will also influence expectations regarding how a person behaves in these family roles.

In addition to our family context, roles reflect our social relations. So we may have roles within our local community (e.g. member of a Neighbourhood Watch scheme), through our sports or leisure activities (e.g. as members of a football team) or as members of a spiritual or religious group. Roles in many of these settings have titles and carry specific responsibilities. For example, committees and societies have a treasurer and secretary and, in work settings, manager, supervisor and team member are common roles (see Box 4.1, overleaf).

In order to take up any role fully and effectively, we need to know what behaviours are associated with the role. Then, we need to look at ourselves

Activity box 4.1 Identifying personal roles

Spend a few moments identifying some of the different family, work and social roles that you have.

Which roles have been given to you and which roles have you chosen yourself?

and see what personal resources we have to bring to the role. Here, personal resources are skills that we have mastered and abilities we have developed over the course of our lives. Taking up a role is partly about trying to match the external expectations with our personal resources.

Figure 4.1 looks at the relationship between skills and abilities and roles. We can see how one individual will have a number of different abilities and skills and may also have a number of roles in their personal, professional and social contexts. Some skills, such as listening, may be used in a variety of different contexts, while others, such as driving and cooking, will be used in fewer settings. In Figure 4.1, we can see that computer skills, patience and an ability to listen would be useful for the role of school governor, whereas cooking and singing may not be any use at all in that role but could contribute to being an effective parent (see also Box 4.2).

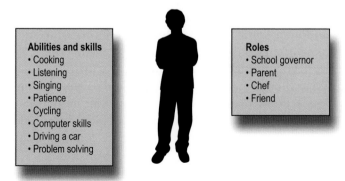

Figure 4.1 An example of abilities, skills and roles.

Activity box 4.2 **Identifying skills and abilities**

Now list some of your own personal skills and abilities and consider which you use in each of the roles you identified in Box 4.1.

ROLES AND THE STUDENT NURSE

Although we may consider being a nurse to be a key part of our identity even when we are not at work (or university), we only assume (or take on) that role in a specific context. Gantt and Agazarian (2005) argue that it is only when we are clear about the context and the goals of the context that we can identify what role we need to take up in order to work towards the goals. Student nurses operate in two different contexts: the university and the practice environment. Here, the term 'practice environment' is used to indicate places where students have the opportunity to gain experience of working with patients, service users, carers and professionals and others. It will include organizations delivering health and social care such as Mental Health Trusts, voluntary organizations as well as primary care. Students may also gain experience in other settings, for example education, training, housing and leisure.

The university and the practice environment have quite different goals. The main goals of a university relate to research, education and training, whereas in the practice environment, the main goal will depend on the organization. For example, the goal of a Mental Health Trust will be to provide mental health care and treatment as the needs of the patient or service user are always paramount. The Trust will often have other goals too that include providing research opportunities or education experiences for student nurses, but these are likely to be secondary goals.

The university

In the UK, nursing is still a relative newcomer to higher education; it is only since the 1990s that all nurse education has been university based. In the

Activity box 4.3 **The role of a university student**

Think about your role as a student and list some of the behaviours associated with the role of being a student in a university. Imagine you are a student on a business or language course, so you can identify the general behaviours associated with being a student rather than being a nurse.

Look back at Box 4.2 and identify which of your personal skills and abilities will be useful in taking up the role of a student.

university context, where research, education and training is the goal, the student's role is to learn (see Box 4.3).

Ability to learn

One of the key requirements of the student role is the ability to learn independently (Marshall & Rowland 1998). In order to do this, the student must master a variety of skills, which include the following.

Reading and making notes

An important aspect of learning is to actively engage with the process. For example, reading a chapter in a book and hoping you will remember the content is a passive strategy. It would be more effective to summarize what you read as you progress through the chapter. Another example of an active strategy would be to discuss what you have read with another student.

Active listening and note taking

In a setting such as a lecture, there is always a tension between listening to the other person and taking notes. Too much note taking can mean missing key points. Again, listening is an active behaviour. A good lecturer should make clear the main issues or themes so that you can then write them in note form. Don't expect to learn everything about a subject from a lecture, but develop taking notes that identify areas that you can follow up later.

Oral skills such as asking questions, participating in discussions and making presentations
Verbal skills are also part of studying and academic development. Most lecturers will be happy to answer questions; you should try to frame your question clearly and concisely. Clarity of focus helps to make a good presentation as well as contributing to useful discussion.

Academic writing
This is partly about being able to communicate ideas clearly for which a good grasp of spelling, grammar and punctuation is necessary. It also requires an ability to handle the content by being able to describe, analyse, critique and synthesize ideas (see Chapter 5, pp. 84–91).

Research skills including the use of information technology
Research skills crucially involve the ability to evaluate the material being discussed or presented. This includes being able to assess whether information is based entirely on opinion or whether there is any evidence in the literature or research to support the ideas.

For further guidance on the learning role, readers are referred to the wide range of study skills books that are available (e.g. Ely & Scott 2006).

The practice environment

The student's role in the university seems clear and straightforward. But what is their role in the practice environment? Remember that the overall goal of this context is to provide mental health care and treatment. The student's primary role is *to learn* about the provision of care and treatment. There are two ways in which the student nurse can take up a learning role: as an observer or as a participant. In the former role, they observe others delivering care and, in the latter, they participate by undertaking to provide some or all of the care themselves under the supervision of a registered nurse. Chapter 3 (Observation) and Chapter 5 (Reflection) discuss the skills that support learning in the practice environment.

A key learning goal for student nurses is to learn about the roles taken on by mental health nurses, as they will need to be able to assume these roles when they become registered nurses themselves. The remainder of this chapter explores these roles but, before doing so, we need to look at the mental health context.

ROLES AND THE MENTAL HEALTH CONTEXT

Until relatively recently, health care was delivered almost exclusively within an institution, and there were clear expectations regarding the behaviour of patients and staff. This included a tendency for patients to be passive and comply with the authority represented by health staff, particularly doctors. There was some merit in this approach as staff had more knowledge about health care and treatment than most patients. Also, being unwell commonly affects concentration and the ability to function to one's full capacity. However, social changes have meant that professionals now have less authority vested in them than was the case previously. Policy is now rightly directing staff towards a partnership approach with individuals receiving health and social care. Patients also have greater access to information, especially through the Internet, and are becoming more knowledgeable, particularly in relation to self-management of chronic conditions.

A contemporary analysis by Quirk (2005) notes the shift away from the total institution described by Goffman (1961) to what he calls 'the permeable institution'. He describes how the boundaries between the institution and the community have become blurred. For example, community staff 'in-reach' to wards by visiting patients when they are in hospital. In contrast, behaviours such as illicit drug use that are common in some domestic environments are imported to inpatient settings as friends of patients see drug use as normal and take drugs into hospital. Mental health staff rarely wear uniform, and it is often commented that, when you go to a ward, it can be hard to tell who are the staff and who are the patients.

Mental health practice is entering a period of significant change. Nurses rarely work in isolation; mental health practice is characterized by a multi-professional approach to patient care. For example, community mental health teams (CMHTs) are usually made up of nurses, occupational therapists, social workers, psychologists and doctors. The importance of creative therapists, including those working in art, music and movement, is increasingly being recognized. A recent proposal by the UK government is the creation of new roles that are not allied to any of the existing professional groups, such as support, time and recovery (STAR) workers. Training is also under way for graduate mental health workers who will work in primary care settings with people with anxiety and depression (Department of Health 2003). At present, these new roles are focusing on primary care with the idea that mental health nurses will focus more on secondary care and people with more complex needs (Department of Health 2006). Currently, there is considerable overlap between the roles of a number of professionals as well as some clear distinctions between them. Roles are becoming more fluid, and established professions such as nursing and medicine must take care to ensure that the roles to which they are attached are responsive to the needs of a modern mental health service.

Roles and the mental health nurse

The roles that mental health nurses have developed have been shaped by a number of factors, including patient needs and expectations, legislation, professional regulation and policy as well as theories of mental health nursing. In practice, nurses have to juggle the different expectations that are made of them. As well as listening to service users, nurses have power and duties under common law in relation to their patients including the duty of confidentiality. Nurses also have a statutory role in administering medication as prescribed by a doctor. There are changes taking place in this area that will give nurses some limited powers of prescription. This is an example of how roles may alter over time.

Service user expectations

Research conducted by service users reported that around half of those interviewed felt they were not getting enough information on a range of issues including their treatment (or clinical issues) and local services (Rose et al 1998). Service users wanted more information about their treatment, such as their medication and the care programme approach, and wanted to be more involved with making decisions about their care and treatment. Many would also have liked information and help with accommodation, benefits and support groups. They also wanted 'someone to talk to' as well as access to non-medication treatments, particularly 'talking therapies'. Mental health services must be responsive to these findings by providing services that fit more with service user expectations.

The Mental Health Act

In relation to legislation, the Mental Health Act (HMSO 1983) invests registered nurses with specific powers including a formal authority to detain patients against their will for a limited period of time and to administer treatment without consent in designated circumstances.

Government policy

In the UK, a number of policy documents relating to mental health have been published recently including the *National Service Framework for Mental Health*

(Department of Health 1999) as well as those relating to occupational standards (see Chapter 1). Although none of the documents specifically identifies roles, they do describe the capabilities that must be reflected in the roles adopted by all mental health professionals. They all emphasize the importance of practising within an ethical framework to work in partnership with individuals, families and communities.

Professional regulation

Professional bodies also influence practice. In 2000, the World Health Organization (WHO) published *Nurses and Midwives for Health: A WHO European Strategy for Nursing and Midwifery Education* (WHO, 2000). The strategy set out a list of principles for initial nurse education that would enable the nurse to undertake five identified roles: care provider, decision maker, communicator, community leader and manager. The Nursing and Midwifery Council (NMC) does not identify specific roles, although it has identified requirements for pre-registration nursing programmes. These are organized into four domains: professional and ethical practice; personal and professional development; care delivery; and care management (Nursing and Midwifery Council 2002). Clearly, there is some overlap between what the NMC are calling domains and what the WHO identify as roles.

Theories of mental health nursing

In the literature, discussion about the role of mental health nurses has traditionally been approached in two ways. First, a discussion about the roles the author thinks nurses should be adopting (or what nurses should be doing) and, second, investigations into what nurses actually do. More recently, Edwards (2005) investigated the role of the nurse by drawing on the views of service users and student nurses to explore what nurses should do, should be and should know. In relation to identifying what nurses should do, Norman and Ryrie (2004) describe two distinct approaches: interpersonal relations and evidence-based practice. In *From Values to Action* (Department of Health 2006), the recent review of mental health nursing, the Chief Nursing Officer of England acknowledged the importance of therapeutic relationships and evidence-based practice.

Interpersonal approach
Peplau is the prime exemplar of the interpersonal approach. In her seminal work on interpersonal relations in nursing, she identified four key roles: teacher, resource person, counsellor and surrogate (Peplau 1952). As a

teacher, the nurse is required to pass on information to the patient, often about health or treatment-related issues including medication, the benefits of exercise or about illness. Being a resource person is also about having information or access to information that the patient does not have; this might include telephone helpline numbers or support groups. Often, the nurse is providing information for services or support that are offered by others, and helping the patient to access these services.

The counsellor role takes a variety of forms. In some contexts, nurses are trained to deliver counselling or psychotherapy, and patients can be referred to these services. Some nurses may also draw upon these techniques in their work with patients. The notion of the surrogate role also has its origins in the psychotherapy literature (notably psychoanalysis). Peplau (1952) is acknowledging that, for some patients, nurses can be seen to represent a significant person from their past; often this person will be a parent. If the nurse does not have some awareness of this process (known as transference), it can make it difficult to have a genuine relationship with the patient in the present as both parties will (usually unconsciously) enact the old roles.

Therapeutic use of self

In these conceptualizations, at the heart of being a mental health nurse is the therapeutic use of self. One of the most important roles that the mental health nurse has, and perhaps the most difficult, is the ability to 'be with' patients and service users. Often, this may mean being with someone during periods of considerable distress. The impact of this on both parties should not be underestimated, and it is for this reason that nursing has been described as 'emotional labour' (Smith 1992).

Evidence-based approach

The evidence-based approach to practice has become increasingly influential, not least because of its inclusion in many of the UK government's recent policy documents. Evaluation and research are essential to the development of evidence-based practice as well as producing evidence from practice. Although a detailed critique is beyond the scope of this book, two points are worth noting. First, there is the question of what counts as evidence. There has been a tendency to assign greater value to research methods such as the randomized controlled trial than to expert opinion including that from service users and carers (Department of Health 1999). Secondly, there are still only a limited number of interventions (apart from medication) that have been evaluated in mental health care. Nonetheless, it is clear that nurses need to take a more active role in investigating their practice.

CORE ROLES

The second approach is to look at what nurses actually do. A recent study by Rungapadiachy et al (2004) interviewed student mental health nurses to explore their perceptions of the role of the mental health nurse. The roles that emerged were broadly similar to those identified in other recent studies.

The roles were:

- administrator, e.g. documentation, liaison between patients and other members of the care team
- agent of physical interventions, e.g. observation and assisting with personal hygiene
- administrator of drugs
- agent of psychological interventions including spending time with patients
- teacher.

Peplau (1994) notes that what nurses do will be related to current definitions of mental health and mental illness. In the UK, this has been shaped by the policy documents noted earlier. We have drawn on these as well as the literature outlined above to identify three core roles:

1. delivering and managing evidence-based care and interventions
2. providing information
3. managing emotions.

Providing information and managing emotions are quite distinct and discrete roles. It is clear that delivering and managing evidence-based care and interventions is a broad category that will incorporate a number of subsidiary components. In Table 4.1, we have identified some of the skills relating to

Table 4.1 Skills required for the core roles.

Delivering and managing evidence-based care and interventions	Providing information	Managing emotions
Observation	Observation	Observation
Communication	Communication	Communication
Reflection	Reflection	Reflection
Assessment	Evaluating information	Identifying emotions (self and other)
Planning		
Implementation	Providing information	Containing emotion
Evaluation	Teaching	

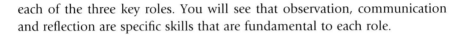

each of the three key roles. You will see that observation, communication and reflection are specific skills that are fundamental to each role.

Delivering and managing evidence-based care and interventions

Care and interventions are outlined in the report entitled *The Capable Practitioner* (Sainsbury Centre for Mental Health 2000) and are organized into the following categories:

- medical and physical care
- psychological interventions
- social and practical interventions
- mental health promotion.

These interventions are explained in Chapter 8.

As noted earlier, at present, the evidence base for some interventions is weak. However, bodies such as the National Institute for Clinical Excellence (NICE) are constantly evaluating treatments and interventions. Therefore, it is important for all nurses to check the current status of interventions they are using. Another source of useful information is the journal *Evidence Based Mental Health* and other mental health or nursing journals.

Managing care includes managing the care you deliver yourself and contributing information to the care team in order for them to make decisions. The final aspect is delegation and supervision of other staff, although this is more relevant to more experienced nurses. Managing care is discussed in Chapter 10.

Providing information

Research into service users' views about the nurse's role (Edwards 2005) found that receiving information was essential to their ability to participate collaboratively in their care. The first annual patient survey (mental health) of over 27,000 patients conducted by the Healthcare Commission (2005: 16) found that 'many service users would like more involvement in decisions about their care and treatment'.

Because of their frequent contact with patients and service users, nurses are ideally placed to provide information about a range of issues. As the amount of information that all of us have access to increases, especially as a result of the Internet, the nurse has a responsibility to know how to access this information. This means becoming familiar with the Internet and search strategies as well as developing an ability to assess the accuracy and usefulness of information. For example, one of the criticisms of the Internet is that many

the reality of the practice of many nurses today. Managing emotions is a component of counselling, and it is something that nurses have to do in the absence of a formal counselling relationship. We believe that the ability to manage emotions may be the most important and the most underestimated aspect of the nurse's role.

The first point to emphasize is that emotions or feelings are a key part of the human experience. When something happens, whether it is a significant event (such as a birth, marriage or death) or a brief exchange in a shop, it is our emotional reaction that affects us and makes us feel happy or sad or sometimes a mixture of feelings. Emotions are a key feature of people's lives as well as thoughts and behaviour. In mental health contexts, we are often working with people who are or have been overwhelmed by their emotions. We can see this with people who are depressed or anxious. Even following a major trauma where someone may be showing little or no emotion, we tend to assume that the emotional impact of the experience has been so great that they have had to shut down their emotions in order to cope.

It can be very difficult being with people who are both experiencing and expressing strong emotions, especially anger and anxiety (Menzies Lyth 1988, Smith 1992). Our work with student nurses also suggests that they can find coping with this work enormously difficult. Although many are resourceful in using staff and other avenues for support, for some, a key strategy is to try and avoid these situations. We believe that this is detrimental to both patients and staff, and that students and staff need access to good supervision and support to manage the work as well as building up a repertoire of skills.

Identifying emotions

Student nurses will have experienced many emotions by the time they come into nursing, but what may be new is beginning to think about emotions. You will learn that, in an extreme form, some of the primary or basic emotions such as happiness, sadness and fear can be characteristics of a mental illness (mania, depression and anxiety). So you will need to learn how to identify emotions in both yourself and others (see Chapter 3, Observation, and Chapter 5, Reflection). By observing yourself and others, you will start to become more aware of the sort of situations that you find most difficult and start to identify patterns regarding your own behaviour, which will most probably be influenced by your emotions.

One aspect of what students find difficult is a feeling of unpredictability about situations and a fear of losing control and being unable to cope. Incidentally, the fear of losing control and not coping is one that nurses share with many patients and service users in situations that are stressful. While it

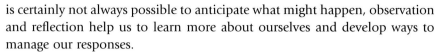

is certainly not always possible to anticipate what might happen, observation and reflection help us to learn more about ourselves and develop ways to manage our responses.

Some emotional responses are predictable in that they relate to specific situations or points of contact, and it is important to be aware of this. For example, apprehension is a normal human reaction to being in a situation that is unfamiliar and, although it may produce some feelings of discomfort, it is not the same as anxiety. In contrast, anxiety is a much stronger emotional reaction that is often fuelled by bodily sensations such as a rapid heart beat or negative predictions about the future such as thinking 'I'm not going to be able to cope with this'. So when people meet for the first time or even at the beginning of a meeting when the people involved have met before, some degree of apprehension is to be expected, and anxiety is not uncommon. Taking care with introductions and explaining the purpose of the meeting will help to manage these reactions (see Box 4.4).

Studies have shown that there is universal recognition of the facial expressions that accompany primary emotions, so you should not have found this activity difficult. However, you will need to remember that some people may

Activity box 4.4 Identifying basic emotions

Think about a recent occasion when you experienced one of the four basic emotions, i.e. happiness, sadness, fear or anger.

Think about what you felt inside and also what others might have seen that would have made them realize you were happy or sad, etc. When thinking about what others would have seen, focus on your behaviour and speech.

Now do the same for each of the other three emotions.

not always be aware of their emotional response or may show a response that is different from what they feel. In addition, people may sometimes conceal their response. For example, a person may feel afraid but does not want to show this. The best way to ensure that you are clear about someone's emotional state or reaction is to ask them how they are feeling.

Containing emotions

Nurses frequently have to contain emotions: both their own and those of the people with whom they work. This is inevitable given that feeling overwhelmed by emotion is often the reason why patients and service users seek help. Nurses must be attuned to the other person's emotional state and demonstrate empathy (often this can be done by listening). It can also be helpful to name the emotion, for example by saying 'I can see you're very upset/afraid' as this also shows that you understand what the person is feeling.

Many of us find it difficult to deal with anger. One of the benefits of taking up a role is that it can help us to take things less personally. Imagine that you have just been shouted at by a patient. If you only take this personally, you are likely to feel angry, hurt or humiliated and experience a strong urge to retaliate; all you will be aware of is yourself and how bad you feel. If you can hold on to your 'nurse' role, you are much more likely to have a sense of the other person and a clearer view of what would be the most appropriate response to the situation.

Dealing with anger

When people feel angry, they often describe taking a deep breath and counting to 10 before responding. In fact, this is a good way to contain the emotions you might be experiencing as well as enabling you to move back into the nursing role. As a student, you should be given or seek support following this sort of incident. Although there are some things you can do on your own, such as reflection or writing in your journal, talking to others is also important. You should be able to learn something about the situation, for example whether the anger seemed to come out of the blue or whether there were signs that you missed.

Self-management

In relation to containing emotion, self-management is essential. Imagine if every time you spoke to someone who was depressed you started crying, or became very anxious when you were with an anxious person. Although this

Activity box 4.5 Personal skills and abilities and the core roles

Look back at Box 4.2 (p. 65). Which of your skills and abilities could you bring to each of the three core roles?

might seem to demonstrate strong empathy, it is unlikely to be perceived as helpful to either person if it happened all the time. Generally, it is helpful for the nurse to mirror the other person's mood state in their behaviour, but usually not to the same degree. So when you are with someone who is depressed, crying is not appropriate, but a solemn or subdued demeanour would indicate being attuned to the other person. It is part of the nurse's role to demonstrate openness, warmth, approachability and a sense of calm. This helps the nurse to contain emotions and helps to contribute to an environment that is perceived as safe and containing by others (see Box 4.5).

SUMMARY

- Becoming a mental health nurse is about taking on the role of the nurse. We can use the skills and abilities we have developed in our personal lives, but will need to decide which of these are relevant to the role.
- We need to be aware of the context in which we are working with patients and service users as this will impact on the goals of care.
- Once we have clarified the context and the goal, it will be easier to decide which role to adopt.
- There are three core roles for mental health nurses: delivering and managing evidence-based care and interventions; providing information; and managing emotions.
- Providing information to patients and service users is essential to enable people to participate in their own care.
- Learning to contain emotions, both our own and those of the people with whom we work, helps to produce a safe environment.

References

Department of Health (1999) *National Service Framework for Mental Health*. London: Department of Health.

Department of Health (2003) *Fast-forwarding Primary Care Mental Health: Graduate Primary Care Mental Health Workers – Best Practice Guidance*. London: Department of Health.

Department of Health (2006) *From Values to Action: The Chief Nursing Officer's Review of Mental Health Nursing*. London: Department of Health.

Edwards K (2005) *Partnership Working in Mental Health Care. The Nursing Dimension*. Edinburgh: Elsevier Churchill Livingstone.

Ely C, Scott I (2006) *Essential Study Skills for Nurses*. Edinburgh: Mosby.

Gantt SP, Agazarian YM (2005) Overview of the theory of living human systems and its systems-centered practice. In: SP Gantt and YM Agazarian (eds) *SCT in Action. Applying the Systems-Centered Approach in Organizations*. New York: iUniverse.

Goffman E (1961) *Asylums: Essays on the Social Situations of Mental Patients and Other Inmates*. Harmondsworth: Penguin.

Healthcare Commission (2005) *Patient Survey Report 2004 – Mental Health*. London: Healthcare Commission.

HMSO (1983) Mental Health Act. London: HMSO.

Marshall L, Rowland F (1998) *A Guide to Learning Independently*, 3rd edn. Maidenhead: Open University Press.

Menzies Lyth I (1988) The functioning of social systems as a defence against anxiety. In: *Containing Anxiety in Institutions*. London: Free Association Books.

Norman I, Ryrie I (2004) Mental health nursing: origins and orientations. In: I Norman and I Ryrie (eds) *The Art and Science of Mental Health Nursing. A Textbook of Principles and Practice*. Maidenhead: Open University Press.

Nursing and Midwifery Council (2002) *Requirements for Pre-registration Nursing Programmes*. London: NMC.

Peplau HE (1994) Psychiatric mental health nursing: challenge and change. *Journal of Psychiatric and Mental Health Nursing* 1 (1), 3–7.

Peplau H (1952) *Interpersonal Relations in Nursing*. New York: GP Putman.

Quirk A (2005) The Permeable Institution – an Ethnographic Study of Three Acute Psychiatric Wards in London. Presentation at LoMHR&D Research Showcase Conference.

Rose D, Ford R, Lindley P, Gawith L and the KCW Mental Health Monitoring Users Group (1998) *In Our Experience. User-Focused Monitoring Of Mental Health Services*. London: SCMH.

Rungapadiachy DM, Madill A, Gough B (2004) Mental health student nurses' perceptions of the role of the mental health nurse. *Journal of Psychiatric and Mental Health Nursing* 11, 714–724.

Sainsbury Centre for Mental Health (2000) *The Capable Practitioner. A Framework and List of the Practitioner Capabilities required to Implement the National Service Framework for Mental Health*. London: SCMH.

Smith P (1992) *The Emotional Labour of Nursing*. Basingstoke: Macmillan.

World Health Organization (2000) *Nurses and Midwives for Health: A WHO European Strategy for Nursing and Midwifery Education*. Copenhagen: WHO.

www.nmc.org.uk

5

Reflection

> *I thought reflection was a waste of time, something you only did when you had to write an essay. But after that day my mentor and tutor were brilliant. They helped me to reflect on what happened, how I felt about it and what I might do differently if it happened again. I feel I've really learnt a valuable lesson.*
>
> Second year student nurse

INTRODUCTION

Reflection has become a key learning tool for practice-based professions such as nursing. Reflection is an active and intentional process that uses thinking in order to learn from experience (Driscoll 2000). This can help nurses develop their practice and may contribute to the development of a knowledge base, which then becomes the basis for future nursing interventions. The Nursing and Midwifery Council (NMC) requires nurses to maintain their professional competence by keeping up to date with current practice (Nursing and Midwifery Council 2004).

In this chapter, we briefly outline the purpose of reflection in practice-based professions such as nursing. We present a rationale for reflection and describe how you can become a reflective practitioner. We look at the use of reflection in other contexts such as enquiry-based learning and supervision. Finally, we look at the relationship between reflection and the other essential skills of observation, therapeutic relationship and taking on different roles.

PRACTICE-BASED PROFESSIONS

Traditional professions such as law and medicine have a knowledge or theory base that informs practice, but practice professions such as teaching and nursing tend to draw on knowledge from other professions. In nursing, this includes psychology, sociology, anatomy and physiology as well as nursing theory. In mental health nursing, biological, psychological and social models help us to understand how the individual is affected when they have a mental health problem. So, for example, if we think about a patient or service user who is depressed, each of these models could explain why an individual becomes depressed, how they are affected when they are depressed and what treatment or interventions may be used to treat or manage depression.

This provides us with a set of generalizations; it is as if all people who are depressed are the same. However, in practice, what we then find is that, although there will be similarities between people who are depressed, there will also be differences regarding how each person is affected when they are depressed. Theories cannot describe all these variations, which is why practice-based professions need a tool such as reflection in order to compare what is found in practice with what is known through existing theory.

Schon's (1983) influential text *The Reflective Practitioner* discussed reflection for practice-based professions and argued that reflection could be used

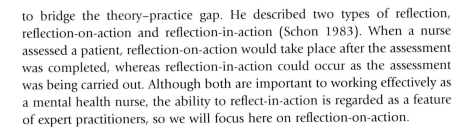

to bridge the theory–practice gap. He described two types of reflection, reflection-on-action and reflection-in-action (Schon 1983). When a nurse assessed a patient, reflection-on-action would take place after the assessment was completed, whereas reflection-in-action could occur as the assessment was being carried out. Although both are important to working effectively as a mental health nurse, the ability to reflect-in-action is regarded as a feature of expert practitioners, so we will focus here on reflection-on-action.

WHAT IS REFLECTION?

Bulman (2004: 4) sees reflection-on-action as the process of 'reviewing experience from practice so that it may be described, analysed, evaluated and consequently used to inform and change future practice'. Reflection allows nurses to look at their practice and understand it within the context in which it occurs. Nurses also compare their practice with others (colleagues, published articles or through research). This may highlight differences between practice and theory. Through reflection, we think about what happens in practice. Often, the focus will be on interaction with a patient or service user, and this can help to make us aware of how we learn. It is part of the process of lifelong learning that allows a nurse to update knowledge and practice skills by integrating experience and knowledge.

The three core components of reflection are practice, the self and theory. Reflection usually begins with something happening in practice, for example an interaction with a patient or service user. Reflection always requires us to think about ourselves and consider our contribution to what is happening in practice. For example, when we talk to a patient, we should be aware of our verbal and non-verbal communication as well as our emotional state. Finally, we can review what happened in relation to theory.

Why reflect?

Reflection can help us to predict what might happen in a specific situation. For example, we may use our experience from having given medication by depot injection to a number of different patients to predict how a woman will react when she is given her first one. When we reflect, we are examining our experiences to see if there is anything to learn that is transferable to other situations that are similar in some way, in relation to:

● another time
● another person.

For example, we could recall occasions when patients had been given a depot injection for the first time and think about how they had reacted. We might have noticed that some were anxious about whether the injection would be painful, and that others were curious about how the medication could be effective over a number of weeks or wondered how long they would have to take it. When thinking about another person, we might consider comparisons with someone who is similar physically or in relation to their lifestyle. For example, if the patient was quite thin, we could think about specific factors that are important when giving an intramuscular injection to a thin person, such as not inserting the needle too deeply.

Mental health care should respond to the changing circumstances of the patient or service user, the context and changes in knowledge. Reflection allows nurses to be flexible in their approach and to adapt to and incorporate changes. Without reflection, care can become automatic and no longer tailored to the individual's needs.

How do we reflect?

We can reflect in different ways at different times. When working with a patient or service user, we can reflect on what is happening between us (reflection-in-action). It is also possible to reflect on the same interaction after it has happened (reflection-on-action). Reflection may be something we do on our own or with others. A number of authors have described models that can be used to structure reflection, including Gibbs (1988) and Johns (1995). Driscoll's 'What? Model' (2000) of structured reflection is similar to Gibbs' in that it provides a learning cycle that can help to guide you through the process of reflection (see Figure 5.1).

You should look at a couple of models and frameworks in order to learn about their similarities and differences. Reflection can also be the basis for other work such as critical incident analysis, clinical supervision, keeping a journal and enquiry-based learning. As a student, it will be helpful for you to follow a model or framework. However, there is also value in developing a habit of reflecting in a less structured or informal way. You can easily do this after an interaction by thinking 'How did that go?' or 'Could I have handled that better?' or 'Why did that work so well?'

BECOMING A REFLECTIVE PRACTITIONER

Reflecting-in-action is rather like having a third eye or ear that sees and hears what is happening and, in order to do this, we need to train the 'observer' part of ourselves. Therefore, as a student nurse, you will find it easier to learn

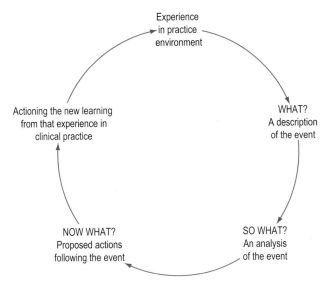

Experience
in practice
environment

Actioning the new learning
from that experience in
clinical practice

WHAT?
A description
of the event

NOW WHAT?
Proposed actions
following the event

SO WHAT?
An analysis
of the event

Figure 5.1 Driscoll's What? model of structured reflection.

to reflect by reflecting on events after they have happened, although there will also be times when you will reflect-in-action as well.

Reflection has become widely accepted in nursing as a method of learning about practice. Despite this, much of the research into reflection in nursing has been relatively small scale (Bulman 2004). Given that it is an important part of nursing practice, it is important to consider how we become reflective practitioners. Atkins and Murphy (1993) undertook a literature review on reflection and identified a number of skills (see Box 5.1). Atkins (2004) notes that, with the exception of self-awareness, all the other skills are also required for academic work and that these higher order cognitive (or thinking) skills may help to integrate theory and practice. Additional skills are also necessary for reflection, including listening, empathy, assertiveness and managing change.

Box 5.1 Skills for reflective practice (Atkins & Murphy 1993)

Self-awareness
Description
Critical analysis
Synthesis
Evaluation

Self-awareness

Self-awareness has long been recognized as essential to the practice of mental health nursing, in which the interpersonal (and therapeutic) relationship is at the heart of the work. For this, we have to observe and know ourselves and have a sense of how we are seen by others. We all tend to have parts of ourselves we know well and other areas that we may not be aware of at all. Who we are is embedded in our values, beliefs and attitudes. It is easy to overlook the impact of our beliefs. This is because we tend to treat our beliefs as if they were facts or universal truths rather than a purely personal view of the world (see Box 5.2).

Beliefs are like 'rules for living' and often have an absolute quality, but they do make it easy to make quick evaluations. We all hold beliefs about ourselves and other people. For example, I may hold the belief that people should be considerate of others or that, in a classroom, students should not talk when someone else is speaking. Beliefs will inform our own behaviour and the meaning we give to the behaviour of others. So, I may keep my music down so that it doesn't disturb my neighbours, and think that they are rude and inconsiderate when I hear their music blaring out. In this example, we can see how beliefs can easily lead to us making value judgements about others. This might then affect how I start to behave; perhaps I might stop talking to the neighbours because I think they are rude.

Another way to identify some of your beliefs is to take a piece of paper and fold it in half. On the left side, write 'I believe I should . . .' and, on the

Activity box 5.2 Identifying beliefs

Think of a recent situation in your personal life (or an item of news) where you found yourself saying 'I can't believe he or she said (or did) that'.

See if you can identify what beliefs underlie your reaction to the other person.

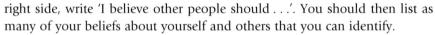

right side, write 'I believe other people should . . .'. You should then list as many of your beliefs about yourself and others that you can identify.

Beliefs are often influenced by gender and culture as well as what are considered to be social norms. They are an integral part of our sense of self, and there is potential for conflict when we are faced with people whose belief systems seem to be quite different from our own. As nurses, we do not have the freedom to withdraw our attention because of our beliefs. Instead, we have to manage our reaction to the difference.

Description

In order to reflect, we need to be able to describe our experience as far as possible by sticking to the facts and leaving aside any judgements or assumptions. In Chapter 3, we outlined how we can use descriptive observation to report and record the appearance, behaviour and speech of others.

As you may discover from the activities in Box 5.3 (overleaf), it can be easy to leave out information that is relevant and include information that is irrelevant, such as judgements and speculations. Remember that a good descriptive account really sticks to reporting or recording what happened, and it will take time and practice to produce this type of description.

It is important to try to reflect as soon as possible after the event, as the more time that passes, the more likely that information will be forgotten. If this is not possible (perhaps you have to finish a shift before you can reflect), try to make some notes to help you recall later. If time is limited, this might involve just noting a few key words that will remind you, for example, of the main facts and feelings.

Critical analysis

Through self-awareness and description, we are largely concerned with identifying the facts and feelings produced by a situation or experience. These provide the basic material for reflection. In the next stage, the aim is to 'unpack' the experience further through critical thinking and analysis. We do this by looking in more detail at each element of the experience.

The word 'critical' needs some comment as it has come to be seen as focusing on the negative. However, in the field of literature, criticism is about taking a much more rounded perspective by examining both sides of an argument, particularly the strengths and the weaknesses. In mathematics and physics, the word critical relates to the transition from one state to another (for example critical mass or critical temperature) and incorporates the notion of transformation. Inherent within the concept of reflection is the idea that we can transform our practice through the process.

Activity box 5.3 Developing descriptive skills

a) Think back to a recent meeting with a friend or family member and write a description of what happened.

b) Now review your description and consider whether it includes relevant information in relation to:
Self: have you recorded your feelings and thoughts?

Others: have you described their appearance, behaviour and speech?

Environment: does the description include information about where you were?

c) Note whether the description includes any information that is not relevant to the account.

Does your account include any judgements or speculation about what happened between you?

The scenario in Box 5.4 is designed to help you explore the different components of critical analysis, which according to Brookfield (1987) are as follows.

Identifying knowledge relating to the situation

It is essential to evidence-based practice that students review experiences to see what (if any) theory or literature might relate to the situation. This can

---

Box 5.4 Scenario for critical analysis

It is your first day on placement in an acute day hospital that provides a group-based programme as an alternative to admission. You have been briefed by your mentor about how the day hospital works and join the community meeting at the beginning of the day.

In the meeting, two patients ask you a number of questions about how long you've been training as a nurse, and whether you've been in an acute day hospital before or worked in groups. You answer each question as honestly as you can and say that you haven't worked in an acute day hospital or had experience of working in groups before. However, you are aware of feeling anxious and uncomfortable about being questioned.

---

help you to understand what happened from a theoretical perspective. In the scenario (Box 5.4), you could identify your knowledge about how groups work as well as ideas about communication.

Exploring feelings and their influence on the situation

Our feelings can have a strong influence on how we function. For example, some people find social situations cause them to feel very anxious, and they may cope with this by avoiding social gatherings whenever possible. Although withdrawal or avoidance is not helpful in the long term, in your personal life, you could decide this is what you want to do. However, now imagine yourself as a student nurse talking to a patient and starting to feel anxious. In your professional role, you do not have the same options as you do in your personal life, so you cannot simply withdraw. Exploring the situation may help you to recognize ways in which you are influenced by your emotions. For example, you might discover that you try to reduce the amount of time you spend with this patient or that you avoid discussing particular topics.

When we have strong emotional reactions, we will probably be aware of how they impact on our behaviour. However, sometimes our responses may be more subtle, and it is through reflection that we have an opportunity to explore the impact of these feelings on our behaviour.

In the scenario (Box 5.4), the student is aware of feeling anxious and uncomfortable, although we don't know whether this feeling is relatively minor or whether it is much stronger. Here, the emotion is clear, but some people find it difficult to identify their feelings, and you may find it helpful to review the section on identifying emotions on p. 76 in Chapter 4. Even in the same situation, it is possible to have different emotional reactions. In the scenario, this might include feeling angry or annoyed with the mentor for not briefing you clearly about what might happen in the group, or feelings of sadness (these might be produced if you make a negative evaluation of your performance).

Identifying and challenging assumptions

In the scenario in Box 5.4, you may be able to identify assumptions that you made when you went into the group, in relation to yourself or the other people. For example, you might have thought that it would not be appropriate for you to bring in your feelings of anxiety and discomfort to the group. You might also have made the assumption that, in the group, the staff would ask the patients questions and assumed that you would not be asked questions, or perhaps assumed that your role was to observe rather than contribute to or participate in the group.

If the assumptions you made regarding how you should behave and how the group would be turned out to be incorrect, the next step is to review your assumptions to determine whether you would make the same assumptions in a similar situation in future. For example, from now on, you might assume that, in another group, the patients might ask you questions. In doing so, you will have altered (and therefore challenged) your existing belief. In relation to some assumptions, such as your role in the group, you might not know whether you should participate in the group and, if so, how best to do this. Here, you should seek guidance from your mentor or tutor as well as seeing whether you can find any literature on this topic.

Imagining and exploring alternative courses of action

Through contemplating alternative courses of action, we can begin to challenge our view that there is only one way that is 'right', and this can help us to develop greater flexibility in our thinking and behaviour. So you could discuss with your mentor how you might have responded to the questions by bringing in some information about how you were feeling. For example, as well as saying that the placement was a completely new experience, you could acknowledge your feelings of apprehension. Many patients can find it helpful when staff report their reactions, as not only is it useful to see how to do this, but it can also make them feel that finding feelings difficult is a universal human experience.

Synthesis

Where analysis is the process of examining in detail (or taking apart) all the components of an experience, synthesis is the opposite; now all the elements are put back together. The aim of reflection is to develop new knowledge, understanding or insight. Sometimes, this is referred to as an 'aha!' experience, when you suddenly understand something. As a student, much of your learning will be at this personal level as you begin to incorporate existing knowledge into your own personal map of nursing.

In the scenario in Box 5.4, there a number of areas where your knowledge and understanding may have altered as a result of reflecting on what happened. For example, you may realize that what happened in the group resulted in your feeling stressed, and this might lead you to think about how a patient feels when they are in a group for the first time. You might realize that, although you had not previously been in a group for patients, you had been in groups while you were at school, and you might look to see whether your reaction was similar in those groups. You might also think about university sessions on the development of groups and think about how to apply these to this situation.

Evaluation

The final and perhaps most important part of the reflection process is to extrapolate what we have learnt from this situation to similar situations in the future. At one level, it is about deciding whether or not we would behave in the same way again. In this context, this is different from evaluating the effectiveness of our actions. Sometimes, we may decide that our actions have met the goal but, nonetheless, in a future similar situation, we would behave in a slightly different way.

As you can see from the example in Box 5.4, it is possible to learn many different things, and these might relate to yourself, to others or to the situation (in the scenario, this is the group or community meeting). It is helpful to the learning process to make explicit what you have learnt. As a student, you are likely to be learning new things all the time, and some of what you become aware of for the first time you will quickly forget as a new piece of learning takes your attention instead.

Evaluation helps to make what we have learned more explicit and makes it more likely that we will retain the knowledge. This is where a reflective journal can be useful, as you can use it to summarize your learning. In addition, you could identify the next steps you could take in relation to areas about which you want to learn more, for example through reading, research or discussion. You could also summarize what you would do in a similar situation in future, such as seeking clarification from your mentor with regard to your role in a situation that is new to you.

TOPICS FOR REFLECTION

Students often wonder what to reflect on, and the answer is everything from the ordinary and everyday to extraordinary or unusual events. As there seems to be so much to learn when you are a student, you may be drawn to reflect on events where you think perhaps you could have done something differently or a situation that went well. As you develop the habit of reflection, over time, you will probably begin to notice some patterns or repetition with regard to your thoughts and feelings. For example, you might become aware of feeling anxious at the beginning of a placement and feeling sad when you are about to leave. You could then make this observation of your own reactions over time the focus of your reflection.

Any aspect of practice can usefully be reflected upon and can provide insight into our own philosophy or approach to care. It is possible to reflect on feelings, thoughts, behaviour, motives, perceptions, attitudes and values.

Reflecting on routines

In nursing, we may regularly repeat certain actions, with the result that they become routine and we no longer consciously think about them. Automatic processes are particularly useful to reflect on in order to avoid the trap of simply carrying out an activity (or task) because 'it's always been done that way'. Reflection helps us look at alternative processes and outcomes. We may look at alternative explanations of the practice situation or issue.

Reflecting on feelings

Reflecting on our feelings and appreciating how others may feel is a way for nurses to develop their emotional intelligence. How we feel both in a situation and after the situation may give us more information about our attitudes, beliefs and values. It may also give us an indication of how the person we are interacting with feels. At times, it can be difficult to separate our own feelings from the feelings produced in us by the other person (this might be a colleague, patient or service user). This is known as countertransference.

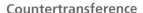

Countertransference

Think of a time when you have been working with someone who was depressed or anxious (patient or colleague). Did you find your mood changing? Picking up on feelings that are not 'our own' can indicate that we are empathizing with others. By reflecting on how we feel, we can examine whether the sadness (or other emotion) is due to the current situation or not. Then we need to ask ourselves if we have felt this feeling before – is the current situation reminding us of previous experiences? If it does, then the feelings may be coming from unresolved issues of our own, and these may need to be addressed through either supervision or counselling.

Dealing with emotions

It is perhaps worth noting that reflection is not a neutral process even though it has the potential to bring many benefits to practice. It is because reflection requires us largely to focus on ourselves and what we thought, felt and did that, at times, it can be painful to do this. This is especially the case when we focus on situations that may have produced a strong emotional reaction.

At times, the emotional experience (often distress) of the patients and service users may become too much to bear and can result in them harming themselves or others. Sometimes, our reaction may mirror (or reflect) the other person's experience, and recalling it in the form of reflection may be painful. In contrast, there will be times when we may block our own emotional responses (particularly guilt, anger, sadness or shame) as feeling them is so difficult. If you have been reflecting on your own and become aware of having a strong reaction, you should seek the support of a mentor or tutor whom you consider will be sensitive to your reactions.

REFLECTION-IN-ACTION

In addition to describing reflection-on-action, Schon (1983) also describes reflection-in-action, although he acknowledges that this is usually a feature of expert practitioners. According to Rolfe et al (2001), most nursing texts have focused on reflection-on-action. Nonetheless, even as student, you will be expected to think about your work with patients as it happens and make adjustments in the light of what you observe.

When we are interacting with another person, we can reflect on the situation by observing how we feel (affect) and our impact on a situation (effect). We use this information to monitor what is happening and to make

newspaper cuttings, drawings and diagrams. In order for this to be a reflective journal, you will need to think about or reflect on what you have recorded. For example, you might keep newspaper cuttings to see how they present issues relating to mental health and illness. The reflection component would require you to think about what you noticed in the reporting.

If you decide to use a more structured approach, as noted earlier, there are many models and frameworks to choose from. A model will help to focus your attention on areas that others have identified as important, and may help you to develop a habit of thinking about areas that you might not necessarily consider.

If you keep a journal, then you will have a permanent record to which you can return. There are some activities in nursing, such as assessment of patients and service users, that you will be involved in repeatedly, and it can be very useful to see how your understanding changes over time. It can also be interesting to see how issues that seemed to be of considerable concern or importance may change over time. A journal may also help you to identify and articulate your learning as you become aware of what you notice in situations that are essentially similar and through seeing how your responses change.

OTHER CONTEXTS FOR REFLECTION

Reflection is a tool for learning that can be used or applied as a 'stand alone' activity' as in a reflective practice session, and it can also be used as a method in other contexts such as enquiry-based learning or clinical supervision.

Enquiry-based learning (EBL)

Enquiry-based learning and problem-based learning (PBL) are examples of learning methods that are student led. Briefly, students are presented with a trigger that contains brief information about a problem or situation (Grandis et al 2005). The student may review what they already know about this subject, and this would include reflecting on their experience, and then use this information to identify their own learning goals. Information on the subject (or problem) can be derived from a range of sources that would broadly include literature (theory and research) as well as practice.

Students often work together to pool their knowledge and make decisions about what else they would like to learn. This is a useful way to learn about a subject and also provides an opportunity for students to reflect on the learning process.

Clinical supervision

Personal development and learning is one of the 10 essential shared capabilities for mental health practice (Department of Health 2004). Clinical supervision is one of a number of methods that qualified staff have for keeping up to date with their practice. It is not the same as reflection but, nonetheless, it does include a reflective component. Supervision can be delivered on a one-to-one basis or in groups, and may be informed by different models or theories. One of the key roles of the supervisor is to facilitate reflection in the supervisee. Usually, this is done by asking the supervisee questions such as 'How did you feel when he said that?'

REFLECTION AND THE ESSENTIAL SKILLS

Observation provides the basic material for reflection as we begin to notice ourselves, others and the environment. In Chapter 3, we note the importance of descriptive observation, which is being able to discriminate between facts or information and judgements or evaluations. Through reflection on your observations, you will become more adept at noticing when you are making judgements and learn about how they may impact on your practice.

The therapeutic relationship (see Chapter 2) is central to working as a mental health nurse. During a placement, you could think about the different relationships you have developed and explore these through reflection. For example, there will be some people with whom you find it easy to form a relationship, and you could consider why this is. The opposite is also true: that you will find it hard to engage with some of the people you meet. Here, you might reflect on how you react when this happens and whether it might affect how you next approach this person.

Peplau (1952) describes relationships as having different stages (such as orientation and identification), and you could reflect on what stage each of the relationships is at. You could consider whether you find it easier to work during some stages rather than others. Through reflecting on different aspects of the therapeutic relationship, the potential for learning is almost unlimited.

You could use a similar approach to exploring the core roles of delivering care, providing information and managing emotion (see Chapter 4). Try to identify a specific situation in which you took on one of these roles. Briefly review or describe what happened and then focus on what you noticed about yourself. Consider whether you feel equally comfortable with each of the roles or if there is one that you find more difficult. When you find something difficult, do you have strategies for helping you to manage the difficulty? Again, there is a potentially rich source of information here.

SUMMARY

- Reflection allows mental health nurses to continue to develop skills, knowledge and emotional intelligence.
- We may choose to reflect on actions, feelings or observations.
- All experiences should be the subject of reflection to improve practice and to celebrate and share good practice.
- Reflection assists us in recognizing learning, processing experiences and determining the appropriate professional response.
- As practitioners, we should be aiming for not just reflection but reflective practice where reflection is integral to all we do.

References

Atkins S (2004) Developing underlying skills in the move towards reflective practice. In: C Bulman and S Schutz (eds) *Reflective Practice in Nursing*, 3rd edn. Oxford: Blackwell.

Atkins S, Murphy K (1993) Reflection: a review of the literature. *Journal of Advanced Nursing* 18, 1188–1192.

Bolton G (2005) *Reflective Practice: Writing and Professional Development*, 2nd edn. London: Sage.

Brookfield SD (1987) *Developing Critical Thinkers: Challenging Adults to Explore Alternative Ways of Thinking and Acting*. San Francisco: Jossey-Bass.

Bulman C (2004) An introduction to reflection. In: C Bulman and S Schutz (eds) *Reflective Practice in Nursing*, 3rd edn. Oxford: Blackwell.

Department of Health (2004) *The Ten Essential Shared Capabilities. A Framework for the Whole of the Mental Health Workforce*. London: Department of health.

Driscoll J (2000) *Practising Clinical Supervision. A Reflective Approach*. Edinburgh: Baillière Tindall.

Grandis S et al (2005) *Foundations for Nursing: Using Enquiry-based Learning*. Basingstoke: Palgrave Macmillan.

Gibbs G (1988) *Learning by Doing. A Guide to Teaching and Learning Methods*. Oxford: Oxford Polytechnic Further Education Unit.

Johns C (1995) Framing learning through reflection within Carper's ways of knowing. *Journal of Advanced Nursing* 22, 226–234.

Nursing and Midwifery Council (2004) *The NMC Code of Professional Conduct: Standards for Conduct, Performance and Ethics*. London: Nursing and Midwifery Council.

Peplau HE (1952) *Interpersonal Relations in Nursing.* New York: GP Putnam.

Rolfe G, Freshwater D, Jasper M (2001) *Critical Reflection for Nursing and the Helping Professions. A User's Guide.* Hampshire: Palgrave.

Schon DA (1983) *The Reflective Practitioner. How Professionals Think in Action.* New York: Basic Books.

Sully P, Dallas J (2005) *Essential Communication Skills.* Edinburgh: Mosby.

Section 2
The process of care

6

Communication

My whole day is spent communicating in one form or another: talking to patients and their carers, making calls to housing and benefit agencies, discussing patient issues with the psychiatrists and social workers, writing letters to GPs, attending meetings about service developments, even having lunch with my colleagues.

Community mental health nurse

INTRODUCTION

Human life is necessarily social. We are surrounded by communication with others, whether family and friends, acquaintances or total strangers. Mental health nursing is an essentially interpersonal occupation. We rely mainly on the basic human channels of interpersonal behaviour and talking together. Clearly, this is a crucial area for mental health nurses as all the essential elements are closely linked with communication. Communication mediates therapeutic relationships and roles, is essential to the process of observation, recording and reporting observations and is key to the process of reflection. Clearly, then, skill in communication is central to the practice of mental health nursing.

This chapter is primarily concerned with communication between the nurse and the patient or service user, their carers and family members and other health care professionals. A definition of communication is provided, and its importance for mental health nurses is discussed. The key aspects of communication to be considered by a mental health nurse are briefly outlined, and a model for appraising verbal communications is presented. Its relevance for each of the four essential skills is then discussed.

THE IMPORTANCE OF INTERPERSONAL COMMUNICATION

Interpersonal communication is the process by which information, meanings and feelings are shared by people through the exchange of verbal and non-verbal messages (Brooks & Heath 1985). Communication may be verbal and face to face or by telephone, or it may be written in the form of letters, reports, care plans or records.

Communication is a key part of a mental health nurse's work, and it is important to be able to communicate effectively. We all bring skills in communication developed in other areas of our lives, but need to develop an awareness of the process and hone our skills, so that we communicate our meaning clearly and easily understand the meanings of others.

Modern mental health care consists of groups of diverse professionals working closely together in multidisciplinary teams. This requires a high degree of communication between professional groups who subscribe to different models of mental health and different ways of understanding the work. These differences provide for important balance between, for example, an overemphasis on disease processes or, alternatively, on social functioning. However, they also introduce a possibility of misunderstanding and conflict, to the detriment of the service. Professionals need to negotiate with each other in order to reach a shared understanding of what is required and to plan suitable care for their patients (Sainsbury Centre for Mental Health 2000).

Nurses hold a pivotal position in the mental health care structure and are placed at the centre of the communication network (see Figure 6.1), partly because of their high degree of contact with patients, but also because they have well-developed relationships with other professionals. Because of this, nurses play a crucial role in interdisciplinary communication. They have a mediating role between the various groups of professionals and the patient and carer (Ritter 1997). This involves translating communication between groups into language that is acceptable and comprehensible to people who have different ways of understanding mental health problems. This is a highly sensitive and skilled task, requiring a high level of attention to alternative views and a high level of understanding of communication.

There is an interaction between our verbal and non-verbal communication. For example, we may reinforce what we say with hand gestures or facial expression, or we may substitute gestures for speech altogether such as a nod of the head meaning 'yes'. There can also be a mismatch (incongruence) between verbal and non-verbal communication, where a person says one thing but their posture and facial expression say something else. For instance, I might say 'I am enjoying myself', but my face shows signs of boredom and my movements are listless and unenthusiastic (Thompson 2002).

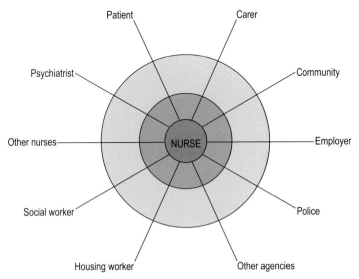

Figure 6.1 Mental health care communication network.

Listening is one of the most important skills because it is through this that we learn about the experience of the other person. We convey that we are listening through our verbal and non-verbal communication.

LISTENING

Although we are all constantly engaged in communicating with others and have a well-developed ability to hear what goes on around us, in ordinary social interaction, we rarely need to listen closely. We are frequently preoccupied with what we are going to say next or distracted by environmental events such as the telephone ringing. In mental health nursing, what is communicated by the patient is of vital importance in gaining an understanding of their internal state and developing a helpful response. Listening, in this context, is an active process, which requires the nurse to suspend their external concerns and focus their attention fully on what the patient is communicating and on the interaction (see Box 6.1).

From the activity in Box 6.1 you may have noticed, for example, that they were doing something else at the same time, such as watching television, or they may have interrupted you and asked apparently irrelevant questions.

In social conversation, we don't usually need to focus our attention on the concerns of the other person in the way that we need to as nurses. We constantly allow our concentration to wander, and this interferes with how we listen. The first step to more effective listening is to begin to notice when this happens. Once you have noticed it, you can refocus your attention and listen to the patient.

 Activity box 6.1 Listening

Think about a recent conversation you had when you thought the other person wasn't listening to you. What did you notice about the other person that made you think they weren't listening?

Obstacles to listening

Hargie et al (1994) identified five obstacles that commonly interfere with listening: divided attention, inattentiveness, individual bias, mental set and blocking.

Divided attention

Divided attention, also referred to as dichotomous listening (Hargie et al 1994: 210), is where the nurse is trying to listen to more than one person or source of information (e.g. telephone, radio, television) at the same time. Their attention and concentration become scattered, resulting in only partial and unsatisfying communication. Sometimes, interacting with a patient in a public space can result in divided attention, and it may be more useful to try and find a quiet and private place to talk. It is also worth noting that patients who are experiencing hallucinations or are very distractible may also have their attention divided.

Inattentiveness

Inattentiveness refers to when the nurse is preoccupied with some concern of their own. This might be to do with the interaction with the patient, for example the nurse may be self-conscious about their performance or nervous about their own safety. On the other hand, the preoccupation may be to do with an external concern such as a domestic problem, a job interview or pressure of work.

Individual bias

Sometimes, in ordinary conversations, we are drawn to an aspect of the other person's subject that is not their main point but, because of our personal bias, is closer to what interests us. For example, John is describing an incident that occurred while he was away on holiday in Spain; Michael is planning to visit Spain on holiday and is interested to ask where John went and how he liked Spain. A similar process can occur between nurses and patients when the nurse is 'caught' by some aspect of the patient's subject that triggers a different train of thought for the nurse. For example, Andrew is talking about an incident that upset him when he was out for a drink with his girlfriend. His community psychiatric nurse (CPN), Clair, points out to him that alcohol interferes with his medication and so he ought not to drink. This might be an important health-promoting point for Clair to make at an appropriate moment, but it does not reflect the distress Andrew is trying to tell her about.

Mental set

This refers to the fact that our attitude to what another person says is often influenced by the preconceived ideas (mental set) we have about that person. For example, a commonly held belief about gay men is that they are indiscriminately promiscuous and sexually irresponsible. Such a belief is likely to interfere with a nurse's ability to listen to a gay male patient talking about his loss of libido as a side-effect of medication. We all have stereotypes and prejudices like this about all sorts of subjects from race, class, gender and religion to more specific ones such as vegetarians or people who wear glasses.

Some nurses harbour stereotypical ideas about people with mental illness or with a specific diagnosis. Preconceptions about a particular patient can also be planted by reading or hearing about the patient's history. If a patient has previously been violent or has a forensic history, for example, although the nurse may need to have this information, they may subsequently filter the patient's communication for evidence of potential violence or criminality, at the expense of listening to the patient's concerns.

Blocking

Blocking refers to a series of techniques that are used to try and avoid some aspect of the patient's communication. These can sometimes be useful, for example if a nurse is having a conversation with a patient in a public place such as a café or watching TV in the ward common room, and the patient approaches personal issues that cannot be safely discussed in that setting, the nurse might employ blocking techniques to steer the conversation back to a topic appropriate to the circumstances. This might involve responding to only the less contentious aspect of the patient's communication or even frankly changing the subject. It is important to be aware that these techniques are also sometimes used by nurses to avoid conversations that they find difficult to deal with. The subject may be deflected or referred (can you talk to your mother about that?) or the nurse might minimize the patient's concern with reassurance (you don't need to worry about that, you'll be alright). Another common method is to restrict the timing or duration of discussions with a patient so that the difficult issue is not brought up in the time or can only be discussed very superficially. If you find yourself using blocking techniques, think about why you are doing this. Is there a good reason, or is the patient trying to raise a topic you are avoiding? Perhaps you need to arrange to give the patient some time and attention in private to discuss the difficult issues (see Box 6.2).

Activity box 6.2 Obstacles to listening

Arrange to observe your mentor talking to a patient and notice their listening skills. See if you notice any obstacles to listening in yourself or the other participants.

Discuss the conversation with your mentor later and refer to the 'obstacles to listening' described in the text.

VERBAL AND NON-VERBAL COMMUNICATION

Interpersonal communication happens through both verbal and non-verbal channels simultaneously. People hold conversations and share information through what they say. But the communication also depends on *how* people speak to each other, for example the tone of voice and how and where they stand or sit while they talk. We all continually monitor both the verbal and the non-verbal communication of the people we interact with but, in ordinary circumstances, our awareness of much of the non-verbal communication occurs below the level of our consciousness so, unless there is something striking about it, we rarely notice it.

As mental health nurses' relationships with patients are mediated through interpersonal communication, it is important to be able understand what they are saying to us, both through the content of their speech and through their non-verbal behaviour. We also need to be able to communicate with our patients in a way that facilitates the therapeutic relationship and helps the patient to feel understood and supported. This means being able to pay attention and listen to both the patient's non-verbal and verbal communication and being able to respond in an appropriate and helpful way.

Paying attention

The first thing required of a nurse is to pay attention to the patient. This means focusing one's mind and listening to the patient, but it also involves expressing interest and support by the way the nurse behaves. If the patient feels that the nurse is interested and paying attention, it makes their interactions more therapeutic, because it becomes easier for the patient to disclose important information and concerns. If patients feel that the nurse is paying attention and taking their concerns seriously, they are more likely to feel that their concerns are serious and to take themselves seriously. This may have benefits for their self-esteem but, importantly, it also makes the patient more likely to approach the nurse with any issues that arise and therefore reduces the risk that they will act on impulse.

Egan (2002) suggests the acronym 'SOLER' as a framework for behaviour which demonstrates that you are paying attention during interactions (Figure 6.2).

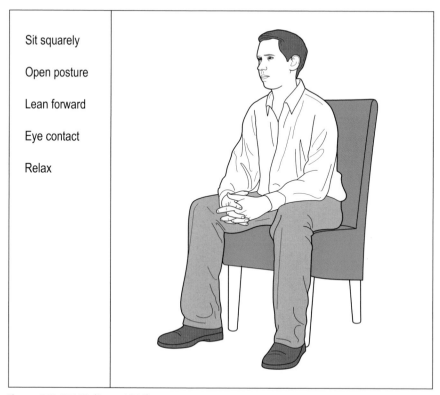

Sit squarely

Open posture

Lean forward

Eye contact

Relax

Figure 6.2 SOLER (Egan 2002).

Sit squarely

Orient your body position directly towards the patient. Turning your back to someone or sitting sideways on to them may indicate that your attention is divided or directed elsewhere, whereas fully facing the patient reduces the likelihood of your attention becoming distracted and indicates that your attention is focused directly on them. This does not suggest a direct face-to-face encounter, which may be experienced as intimidating or aggressive but, even when the seating is arranged at an angle to the patient, your body can be positioned squarely towards the patient.

Open posture

An open posture is one that leaves the 'vulnerable' parts of the body open and unobstructed by arms, legs or hands. This suggests that the listener is receptive to the other person's communication and prepared to allow it to 'touch' them, rather than defending themselves against it by using limbs as deflecting barriers. This means avoiding folding arms across your chest or crossing your legs, as well as keeping your hands away from your face and mouth so your expression can be clearly seen and what you say can be heard.

Lean forward

People who are having intimate conversations often lean slightly towards each other. This has the effect of bringing their heads more closely together so they can see and hear each other easily. It also reduces the distractions in their peripheral vision and makes their conversation less accessible to outsiders. It is important, however, to be aware of an appropriate personal distance between you, as coming too close to the person can also be experienced as intrusive and intimidating. This can be judged by observing the patient's response. If you are too close to them, they will tend to move back; if you are too far from them, they may try and move closer.

Eye contact

The maintenance of steady eye contact indicates that the listener is engaged in the conversation. Eye contact levels fluctuate from moment to moment during the course of a conversation but, in general, in western and European cultures, a person looks attentively at the other when they are listening, but may glance away more frequently when actually speaking. Eye contact is a very important feature of communication as we unconsciously monitor the involuntary dilations and contractions of the other person's pupils, allowing us to gauge their interest in our conversation. It also plays an important role in alerting us to when the other person has stopped and it is our turn to speak.

Relax

This requires the nurse to become comfortable with adopting the other behaviours described here, so they are not preoccupied with their external behaviour, but are able to relax and focus their mental attention on the patient. It also involves avoiding distracting fidgeting and grimacing.

Cultural issues

The SOLER framework can be used as a general guideline, but should also be used with caution, as some of these behaviours may vary between cultures. For example, different cultures have different norms about the distance it is comfortable to maintain between oneself and a person you are speaking to socially. Also, in some cultures, it is important to maintain steady eye contact while speaking, but a sign of listening would be the avoidance of eye contact. In a multicultural society, it is impossible to anticipate the cultural norms of all the patients you might encounter, but it is important at least to have an awareness of the behavioural expectations of the major local populations, and to be aware that your behaviour may have a different meaning from what you intend when interacting with a patient whose culture is unfamiliar to you. It may be appropriate to discuss this with them and their carers and to try and adopt behaviours that help them to feel socially at ease and trusting with you.

Non-verbal communication

Mental health nurses need to develop the skill of attending to their patients' non-verbal communication, sometimes called 'body language', in order to understand as fully as possible what the patient is communicating. Bull (2001) suggests that the main role of non-verbal communication is to express emotions, which may not necessarily be expressed verbally. From the point of view of the nurse, it is important because it allows you access to the patient's inner experience, which may not be accessible through their speech. If the patient is not speaking, their non-verbal behaviour will help the nurse to make some inference about their emotional state. If the patient is also speaking, it is the relationship between the content of their speech and their non-verbal behaviour that is most revealing.

Egan (2002), echoing the work of Knapp (1978), outlines four ways in which non-verbal communication can relate to speech.

Confirming or repeating

What the patient says may be echoed in their non-verbal behaviour, thus confirming the verbal message. For example, a patient telling a nurse they are looking forward to a visit from their family may smile broadly with raised eyebrows and speak in an animated way at a slightly higher pitch. They may also adopt a relaxed and open posture and engage in steady eye contact.

Denying or confusing

The non-verbal behaviour, on the other hand, might contradict or confuse the patient's verbal message. For example, the patient who says they are looking forward to a family visit may speak in a monotonous, perhaps a tremulous, voice and may have a blank or serious expression. Their posture may be stooped with hands or arms across the body and they may avoid eye contact.

Strengthening or emphasizing

The patient's verbal message may be reinforced by being accompanied by non-verbal behaviour that underlines the emotion expressed. For example, the patient telling the nurse they are really looking forward to the family visit may emphasize the strength of their feeling by changing the pitch and volume of their voice as they say 'really', and by nodding their head and making hand gestures at the same time.

Controlling or regulating

Non-verbal cues play an important role in regulating interpersonal communications. On p. 114, we mentioned how eye contact helps to indicate turn taking in speech, but other behaviours also play important roles. For example, someone who wishes to end a conversation may break eye contact and turn their body slightly away from you.

Interpreting non-verbal communication

Although a person can manipulate their non-verbal behaviour, it is less consciously controlled than speech and so may provide a more direct and reliable version of the patient's state. Where there is some uncertainty, for example where the non-verbal and verbal messages are contradictory, it may be helpful to clarify with the patient. For example, if the person's non-verbal behaviour appears to contradict what they are saying (see 'Denying or confusing' above), the nurse might say 'although you tell me you are looking forward to the visit, you look a bit worried about it', giving the patient the opportunity to clarify the contradiction and to explore their feelings more searchingly.

Non-verbal behaviour

Argyle (1994) provides a useful guide to the channels and locations of non-verbal behaviour (Figure 6.3).

Facial expression

Most people display their emotions through the expression on their face. Argyle (1994) suggests there are six basic emotional expressions:

- happiness
- surprise
- fear
- sadness
- anger
- disgust.

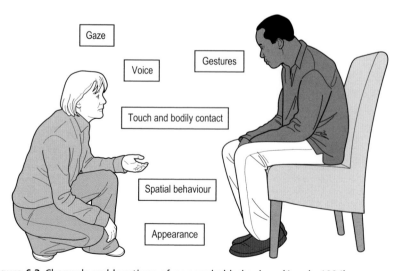

Figure 6.3 Channels and locations of non-verbal behaviour (Argyle 1994).

When we communicate, we tend to look at our companion's face and read their expression unconsciously. Of course, it is possible to disguise one's emotions by adopting an alternative facial expression, such as 'smiling through adversity'. We also use our faces to illustrate and emphasize the content of our speech.

Gaze

The direction of a person's gaze gives a strong indication of their emotional state. Someone who is feeling sad, for instance, may direct their gaze downwards or, if they are preoccupied, they may 'gaze into space'. On the other hand, someone who is feeling cheerful and confident may maintain a steady gaze ahead, 'look the world in the eye' so to speak. This is also the case with interpersonal eye contact; someone who is feeling happy is more likely to initiate and maintain steady eye contact, whereas someone who feels sad or afraid may avoid eye contact.

Voice

The way a person speaks, as opposed to what they say, is also a powerful aspect of their non-verbal behaviour. The tone and pace of their speech reveals different emotional states, for example someone who is excited may speak loudly and quickly, while someone who is angry may shout.

Gestures

People constantly accompany their speech with movements of their hands, body and head, which serve to emphasize and illustrate the content of the speech. However, gestures may also provide information about the emotional state of the person, for example clenched fists may indicate anger, or someone who is anxious may touch their face. Some gestures also have specific meanings and may replace speech altogether, for example a nod of the head indicates agreement or assent and a wave of the hand indicates a greeting.

Posture

The way a person carries their body or stands may be habitual or may indicate a physical injury; some people habitually walk in a slightly stooped posture, for example. However, a person who is feeling happy and confident is likely to adopt a more erect posture with square shoulders and their head held high, whereas someone who feels sad or disappointed may allow their head to hang forward and their shoulders and back to slump forward into a slouch.

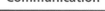
Touch and bodily contact

Touch is a very powerful vehicle for the expression of emotions such as affection and hostility and should be approached with caution by nurses. People who feel affectionate towards each other may touch each other frequently. The areas of the body that can be touched will depend on the type of relationship, with intimate areas being reserved for close, usually sexual, relationships. Except when the nurse is providing personal care with the consent of the patient, intimate touching between nurses and patients should be avoided as it may be interpreted as sexual, or at least as intrusive. However, patients may wish to hold or touch your hand when they are distressed and may express aspects of their emotional state through variations in the pressure of touch.

Spatial behaviour

Spatial distance refers to the distance between us and other people. We all have a social distance at which it is comfortable for us to communicate with others. The distance varies a little, depending on our relationship with, and feelings about, the person we are speaking to. We may move closer to someone we know well and are fond of, and maintain more distance with someone we have just met or are suspicious of. A person's physical orientation towards or away from you also indicates their attitude to you and to the conversation you are having. A person who is uncomfortable or uneasy is likely to turn away slightly, whereas a person who is deeply interested in the conversation is likely to turn squarely towards you.

Appearance

Clothes and style of dress and hair indicate the person's status and role, for example whether a man wears a business suit or a boiler suit, but they can also communicate suggestions about the person's emotional state, for example a person who is dressed in fashionable or revealing clothes for a meeting with their community nurse may be expressing something about their feelings towards the nurse, or they may have a generally good feeling about themselves, or they may even feel generally aroused. Equally, a person who is feeling listless and lethargic may not take much care with their appearance.

Cultural issues and non-verbal behaviour

Non-verbal behaviour can be ambiguous. People have different understandings of social cues according to their social and cultural background, and so your interpretation of particular behaviours may not correspond with theirs. For this reason, it is important to treat your observations with caution and to understand them in the context of the content of both the patient's speech and the conversation generally.

Self-awareness of non-verbal behaviour

It is also worth remembering that, when you are in contact with a patient, while you are appraising their non-verbal behaviour and communication, they are doing the same to you, although this may be less consciously and therefore less purposeful. It is important as a mental health nurse to have an awareness of the messages you are communicating to your patients generally through your appearance and behaviour, and to be conscious of the professional standards required of you. It is particularly important to have an awareness of your non-verbal communication in an interaction with a specific patient as the therapeutic relationship (see Chapter 2) is developed and maintained by the quality of communication between you.

HERON'S SIX-CATEGORY INTERVENTION ANALYSIS (HERON 2001)

Heron's six-category intervention analysis is a system for analysing verbal interventions into categories. It is not a model for therapeutic interventions; rather, it describes six basic intentions that a nurse may have in verbal communication. Heron (2001) is concerned with therapeutic communication in the context of 'helping relationships'. The framework can also be useful when deciding what to say and how to respond and when analysing professional communication.

Heron (2001) suggests that finding the words to say something follows from identifying what it is you intend to achieve by what you say, i.e. what your intention is. So, it is similar to framing a question that is likely to elicit the sort of information one wants. Heron's six-category intervention analysis helps the speaker to frame an intervention or to say something that matches what they hope to achieve by saying it.

Importantly, Heron (2001) is not suggesting that there is a formula for finding the 'correct' form of words. As he points out, interventions occur in relationships, and the variations in the use of words depend on who the participants are and what is happening between them.

Authoritative–facilitative continuum

Heron (2001) identifies two main types of intervention, authoritative and facilitative, which occupy opposite arms of a continuum relating to underlying

Heron's six-category intervention analysis (Heron 2001)

Authoritative	Facilitative
Assumes high degree of knowledge and authority located in speaker	Assumes hearer has knowledge and autonomy

Figure 6.4 Continuum of authoritative and facilitative interventions (Heron 2001).

assumptions about the locus of knowledge and authority in a relationship or interaction (see Figure 6.4).

The two types of intervention are each divided into three categories, making a total of six categories.

Authoritative interventions

The authoritative interventions are more hierarchical, in that the nurse carries responsibility in the form of authority and knowledge, about what is best, about a specific subject or about the patient's behaviour. There are three categories of authoritative intervention: prescriptive, informative and confronting.

Prescriptive interventions

The intention of a prescriptive intervention is to overtly or covertly influence and direct the patient in a course of action or behaviour. There is an assumption that the nurse is in a better position to evaluate a course of action or behaviour and therefore carries authority.

Example: The nurse makes a suggestion to the patient about the structure of their day: 'try making an arrangement to meet someone in the morning to give you a reason to get out of bed'.

Informative interventions

The intention of an informative intervention is to provide knowledge or information to the patient. The assumption here is that the nurse has knowledge or information that would be helpful to the patient. It is also assumed that the patient would be able to evaluate this knowledge or information.

Example: The nurse provides the patient with information about the therapeutic action of their medication: 'the antidepressant the doctor has prescribed usually starts to have an effect about 10 days to 2 weeks after you start taking it'.

Confronting interventions

The intention of a confronting intervention is to point out to the patient (in a helpful way) some inconsistency in an aspect of themselves that is critical

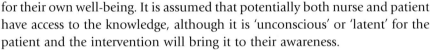

for their own well-being. It is assumed that potentially both nurse and patient have access to the knowledge, although it is 'unconscious' or 'latent' for the patient and the intervention will bring it to their awareness.

Example: The nurse challenges the patient's assertion that there is nothing wrong with them by pointing out that they have engaged voluntarily in treatment: 'on one hand, you have told me that you don't think there is anything wrong with you, but on the other hand, you have agreed to the treatment that has been prescribed. I wonder why that is?'

Facilitative interventions

The facilitative interventions assume that the patient retains responsibility and autonomy and is able to be knowledgeable about a specific subject, about themselves and about what is best. These interventions are cathartic, catalytic and supportive.

Cathartic interventions

The intention of a cathartic intervention is to enable the patient to come into contact with (abreact) painful emotion from which they have shielded themselves. It assumes that the nurse is aware of the presence of emotion, and that the patient is able to know about it and to cope with that knowledge.

Example: The nurse gently points out the unnamed emotion suggested by a patient's verbal or non-verbal communication: 'you seem quite sad about this'.

Catalytic interventions

The intention of a catalytic intervention is to facilitate new self-understanding or discovery in the patient. The assumption is that the patient can accept their own responsibility, and can access a deeper level of self-knowledge if the nurse plays the role of catalyst.

Example: The nurse reflects (repeats back), without implying either a question or agreement, a significant word or phrase contained in the patient's speech.

Patient: 'I find it hard looking after a family on my own, I want another parent, there's all the practical stuff to manage, like shopping, and all the other support and encouragement as well. It's hard to do it all on my own.'

Nurse: 'You want another parent'.

Supportive interventions

The intention of a supportive intervention is to validate the patient's self-knowledge and self-responsibility. It assumes that the patient is responsible for themselves, and that the patient is also knowledgeable about themselves.

Example: The nurse acknowledges the patient's ability to make their own decisions: 'you don't seem to agree with what I suggested so you must have your own thoughts about that'.

Using Heron's six-category intervention analysis

Heron's (2001) six-category intervention analysis is useful for mental health nurses in making choices about what to say in a given situation. Although most of us are able to 'get by' in our personal lives, we all have experience of speaking without thinking and, sometimes, that has undesired consequences. In our working lives, we have specialized professional and therapeutic relationships in which communication requires a higher level of skill. Heron (2001) provides a useful framework for helping you to select a form of words according to your intention in making the intervention. It is also useful to use the tool in reflecting on your interactions as a way of assessing your performance against your intention, and thinking about what you might have said to more closely match your intention.

COMMUNICATION AND THE ESSENTIAL SKILLS

The therapeutic relationship can only be built on a foundation of effective communication skills. Listening is the most important element, as it is through this that we learn about the other person and, by active listening, that we convey that we are interested in what they are saying.

Communication and the therapeutic relationship

Within the therapeutic relationship, nurses can also explore how the patient communicates with them and with others. For example, the nurse might raise the issue of communication and get the patient's agreement to discuss this, as they have noticed that the patient rarely initiates a conversation or that they easily get into disagreements with others.

Communication and observation

Observation relates to self, others and the environment, and each element should be considered to ensure that communication is effective. It is easy for nurses to focus on patients and service users and observe their communication. However, we also need to be able to hold a mirror up to ourselves in order to understand how we might be perceived. For example, sometimes shyness can be perceived as being aloof and uninterested even though this is not the intention. Patients do not always feel able to give direct feedback to nurses, but they will act on their perceptions. This is where reflecting on communication is an extremely useful learning tool.

Observing the other person's verbal and non-verbal behaviour also provides information that can be used to help to decide what type of response to make. For example, a confronting intervention can be used to draw attention to the discrepancy between what the person is communicating verbally and their non-verbal behaviour.

Communication and roles

Communication is also important in relation to the different roles, i.e. delivering care and interventions, providing information and managing emotion. The care and interventions that nurses provide have physical, psychological and social elements. The general aspects of communication include providing an explanation to the patient in order to enable them to participate in their care. At times, the nurse will also provide specific information such as how to manage anxiety. Providing information is discussed more fully on p. 195. The final role relates to managing emotions by identifying and containing them. Nurses must learn to manage their own emotions. At the same time, they also need to be able to communicate their emotional reactions to the patient, albeit in a modified form.

SUMMARY

- Listening is one of the most important skills because it is through this that we learn about the experience of the other person. We convey that we are listening through our verbal and non-verbal communication.
- Listening is an active process that requires the nurse to attend to what the other person is communicating.
- Obstacles to listening include divided attention, inattentiveness, individual bias, stereotyped views of people and blocking.
- Communication includes verbal and non-verbal elements.
- Egan (2002) uses the acronym SOLER to describe behaviour that demonstrates that you are paying attention to the other person.
- Heron (2001) has developed a system for describing verbal interventions based on their underlying intention or purpose.
- Heron's six-category intervention analysis is useful for mental health nurses in making choices about what to say in a given situation.

References

Argyle M (1994) *The Psychology of Interpersonal Behaviour.* London: Penguin.

Brooks W, Heath R (1985) *Speech Communication.* Dubuque, IA: WC Brown.

Bull P (2001) *Communication Under the Microscope.* London: Routledge.

Egan G (2002) *The Skilled Helper: A Problem–Management and Opportunity–Development Approach to Helping,* 7th edn. Pacific Grove, CA: Brooks/Cole.

Hargie O, Saunders C, Dickson D (1994) *Social Skills in Interpersonal Communication.* London: Routledge.

Heron J (2001) *Helping the Client: A Creative Practical Guide,* 5th edn. London: Sage.

Knapp M (1978) *Nonverbal Communication in Human Interaction,* 2nd edn. New York: Holt, Rinehart and Winston.

Ritter S (1997) Taking stock of psychiatric nursing. In: S Tilley (ed) *The Mental Health Nurse: Views of Practice and Education.* Oxford: Blackwell Science.

Sainsbury Centre for Mental Health (SCMH) (2000) *The Capable Practitioner. A Framework and List of the Practitioner Capabilities required to Implement the National Service Framework for Mental Health.* London: SCMH.

Thompson N (2002) *People Skills.* Basingstoke: Palgrave.

7

Assessment

Assessment is the main tool for finding out about the patient's needs. I need to remember that we work with people, not problems.

Second year student nurse

INTRODUCTION

Assessment is woven into our lives in different forms. As we cook, we check the flavour of the food to see if more seasoning is needed. In the garden, we consider factors such as the weather to decide if it is the right time for planting. We also assess when we notice that something is not as we think it should be, for example noticing a leak in a water pipe or a strange noise in the car engine. We may debate whether this poses a risk (perhaps the leak is near an electrical cable) and whether or not we can deal with the problem. If we do not have the relevant knowledge, we will probably have to call someone in to assess the problem and suggest some solutions. These relatively simple examples of assessment incorporate a problem-solving approach and the notion of an external person (often identified as an expert) brought in to manage or solve the problem. Implicit too, as Barker (2004) notes, is the idea that we assess in order to make decisions about what actions to take in the future.

The focus of nursing is helping the individual to manage the dynamic between health (and well-being) and illness. In this chapter, assessment is seen as a process rather than a 'one-off' activity. It begins with identifying the context and goals of assessment. We identify three areas to assess: strengths, physical and mental health, and risk. This is followed by methods of assessment with particular emphasis on the interview. Finally, we discuss how the four essential skills relate to the assessment process.

THE ASSESSMENT PROCESS

Assessment should be seen as an ongoing activity rather than a single or one-off event, which is why we describe it as the assessment process. Assessment can be a formal, structured process, such as takes place when a patient is first admitted to hospital, but nurses also make informal assessments of patients and service users whenever there is contact between them. Before undertaking any assessment, there are a number of factors that need to be considered, including the ethical aspects, models of assessment, the context and the goals of assessment. Thinking about each of these areas helps us to plan more precisely the type of assessment we want to conduct.

Ethical aspects of assessment

In order to practise ethically, it is necessary to think carefully about the care that is being delivered, particularly with a view to identifying areas where ethical issues are most likely to arise. For example, the interview is commonly used to gather information for assessment. Many of our questions focus on areas that are distressing to patients and require them to reveal information about behaviours that may be illegal or potentially criminal (for example, the use of illicit drugs or violence to others). This touches on two important areas: maintaining confidentiality and seeking only information that is relevant to the situation.

Maintaining confidentiality

Patients need to know what will happen to the information that they provide. The nursing code of professional conduct provides guidance regarding the issue of confidentiality (Nursing and Midwifery Council 2004). Although nurses have a professional obligation to maintain confidentiality, in practice, information about patients is often held by or shared between a team of professionals including the patient's general practitioner. Patients may not always be aware of the number of people who are entitled to access information about them.

Seeking only information that is relevant

The second important point is that, as professionals, we are in a privileged position in having access to information about the patient that they might sometimes prefer to withhold. We can view this as an informal contract whereby the patient agrees to co-operate and provide information. The nurse's responsibility is to seek only information that is relevant.

Models and conceptual frameworks

One way to help make decisions about the content of the assessment process is to use a model or conceptual framework. Examples of models that are frequently used in mental health include nursing models, medical models and psychological models. In broad terms, nursing models are derived from beliefs about nursing, whereas medical models are rooted in biological concepts of illness and disease within the body. Psychological models help us to understand individual functioning, and social models look at the individual within the context of his or her social environment.

Each category may include a number of different models based on inherently different theories. For example, among the psychological models, the cognitive behavioural model and the psychoanalytic model have quite different views on individual functioning. Nursing models may be organized

Looking at the brief scenarios in Box 7.1, Solomon and Mary and their families as well as John are likely to be experiencing some degree of apprehension as they enter a period of change and uncertainty. Apprehension is a normal reaction to the unknown and brings in its wake some discomfort. Anxiety, on the other hand, is a much stronger emotional reaction that is often fuelled by bodily sensations such as a rapid heart beat or negative predictions about the future, such as thinking 'I may never get over this.' In contrast, we might suppose that Amira may not experience any apprehension, let alone anxiety, as she is in a situation that is very familiar to her. However, it is worth remembering that, although we can always guess how people are reacting to the situation in which they find themselves, we can never be sure unless we ask them.

In many states where a strong emotion such as anxiety, anger and depression or elation is present, the predominant mood state can affect concentration and attention. We can use this awareness to ensure that we try to work to a timeframe that increases the likelihood of people being able to concentrate and co-operate. For example, this might mean introducing breaks or shortening the assessment process as well as taking care to ask questions as clearly as possible.

Goals of assessment

Before formally embarking on the assessment process, we should ask ourselves 'what is it that I want to do?' Barker (2004) captures what he perceives to be the essence of the work in the phrase 'In search of the whole person', which he uses as a subheading for his seminal text on assessment. In nursing as well as in medicine, assessment has often focused on problems. Although there are valid reasons for this, especially in emergency situations, this approach has undoubtedly contributed to the power imbalance between patients and staff. It is important to remember that, as mental health nurses, we work with people not problems. Contemporary approaches to care (in part influenced by the views of service users) require that we take a much broader approach to assessment than simply focusing on problems and needs.

The goal of assessment is to obtain information about the individual in relation to three key areas:

- their strengths
- their physical and mental health
- risk.

The order of assessment of these areas will vary depending on the context. Look back at Box 7.1 and consider which of these areas is likely to take precedence within the contexts described.

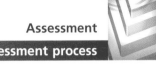

In relation to Solomon, who is being assessed in an accident and emergency department, assessment of his mental health would be a priority. This in itself could give information about issues of risk. For example, if Solomon described not sleeping properly, starting to hear voices and beginning to think that his father might want to kill him, the nurse would explore this further to see if there is a risk of Solomon harming his father or himself as a result of what is happening to him.

With Mary, her physical and mental health will be a priority. We already know that her husband is worried about her safety so would want to find out more about this. He might describe how she forgets to turn the gas off on the cooker and has sustained burns to her hands as the gas flares when she lights it later. She might also forget to eat and drink and physically be in poor health.

Amira meets her CPN regularly, and this would be an ideal context to assess her strengths. However, if Amira is depressed, it is likely that her view of herself will have a negative bias, and she may find it difficult to recall or identify more positive aspects of herself. It would also be important to know about John's strengths as these would help him in the process of being rehabilitated back into the community. As he is being nursed in a secure setting, assessment of risk will be a high priority, but it is important that other aspects of his life and functioning are included.

Strengths assessment

Rapp (1998) describes the strengths model as a paradigm shift within the helping professions. Although his account refers particularly to the development of social work, it has relevance for nursing, which, like medicine, has been dominated by 'clinical diagnosis (that) focuses on a human lack or weakness' (Rapp 1998: 3). Nursing, along with other disciplines, has tried to move away from medical models towards a problem-solving approach. However, Rapp (1998) contends that this is still characterized by an emphasis on what the person is unable to do.

In contrast, strengths models aim to build a different profile of the individual, one that is not rooted in illness and problems. For nurses, this means exploring with the person their abilities, interests and resources. It may be helpful to consider abilities and interests as being located within the individual whereas resources are external.

Abilities

Consider what skills or abilities the person has. These might relate to interpersonal skills such as listening as well as practical skills including being able to drive or cook or the ability to use IT equipment.

Interests

Find out what interests the person. Do they have general interests such as watching TV or more specialized interests, for example photography or languages? Are they able to follow these interests currently and, if not, what stops them?

Resources

This refers to what the person has access to and includes people and finances as well as access to facilities and services. In relation to people, the emphasis is on those who are perceived as having a positive impact on the individual (in effect, providing social support). The contact may be face to face, via the telephone or even email; the essential point is whether they have someone to talk to or turn to. Other interpersonal resources may include a sense of belonging through being a member of a church or religious group, or having peers on a course or being part of a group that has shared interests. Financial resources are important, and having an income, probably through either employment or the benefit system, is crucial to most people's well-being.

Undertaking a strengths assessment

When undertaking a strengths assessment, the nurse should aim to elicit information about each area. Some people will find it relatively easy to identify their abilities and interests while others will find it more difficult. The nurse should think about whether the patient or service user is experiencing symptoms that might impact on their ability to access this information. These might include negative thinking, hallucinations, sleep disturbance or concentration difficulties. The duration and content of sessions should be tailored accordingly, and it may be more feasible to develop a strengths profile over time rather than in a single session. If the person is unable to identify any abilities or interests in the present, asking them to think about the past, for example when they were a child or at school, may help them to recall former interests. Family members may also be able to help to build up the profile. Information from the strengths profile can be used to develop a care plan.

Physical and mental health

This is potentially an enormous area, and using a model such as a cognitive behavioural approach to assess these areas can give a clearer focus. It is also important to consider who else may have assessed the patient and what form their assessment has taken. For example, a psychiatrist would normally assess

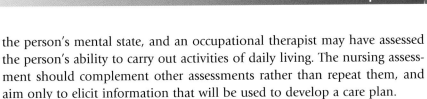

the person's mental state, and an occupational therapist may have assessed the person's ability to carry out activities of daily living. The nursing assessment should complement other assessments rather than repeat them, and aim only to elicit information that will be used to develop a care plan.

Problem-based approach

Assessment often begins by asking the person to outline the problems or difficulties they are currently experiencing. This list can often be very broad and may include issues relating to finances (e.g. claiming benefits), accommodation (e.g. having noisy neighbours) and employment (e.g. returning to employment or training following a period of illness), as well as issues directly related to illness, such as feeling depressed. A broad list gives more information about the contexts in which the person lives. Once a list has been developed, each problem or issue can be explored in more detail. In part, this will provide more information to help the nurse decide whether they can help the person or whether input or advice from a specialist is required. It may also begin to clarify whether there is any relationship between the different problems.

Cognitive behavioural approach

A number of problems or symptoms, such as anxiety, depression and psychosis, can be assessed using a cognitive behavioural framework (Grant et al 2004). This involves examining a specific situation in detail to identify the individual's affect, behaviour and cognition.

Affect
Here, affect is used to represent mood and emotion. How would the person describe their mood? Do they feel happy or sad or anxious? Does what you notice about their mood match how they report feeling?

Behaviour
Is the person aware of any changes in their behaviour or normal routine? For example, they may report that they have they stopped going to the shops because they feel anxious. Conversely, they may describe an increase in some behaviours; they may have started vomiting after eating because they feel fat, or repeatedly checking that the front door is locked when they leave home.

Cognition
The term cognition refers to a number of mental processes including the content of thoughts as well as thought processes. The nurse should check whether the person is aware of any particular types of thoughts, for example

worrying thoughts about what might happen in the future or negative thoughts such as thinking that they don't have a future. Some people report having bizarre or unusual thoughts that they find disturbing. Commonly, such thoughts contain violent or sexual content.

Questioning around thought processes would involve finding out whether the person was having difficulty concentrating. Other aspects to consider are whether the person reports any changes to their thinking processes, for example thinking that thoughts are being taken out of their head or thoughts that are not their own are being put into their head. As our thinking is usually reflected in our speech, the nurse may notice that some patients are speaking very quickly in response to having lots of different thoughts or ideas. In contrast, others will have little to say, as if their thinking processes have almost stopped.

Personal history

By adopting a problem-solving approach, the nurse can ask the patient or service user to provide two types of personal information. The first is information that they think may be relevant to the problems they have described. This helps to provide a focus and makes it less likely that the nurse will be gathering information that will not be used. Once the patient has done this, the nurse can ask whether there is anything else about themselves that they would like the nurse to know. This can be helpful in developing a partnership approach, as it gives the patient more control over the information they wish to disclose.

Family history

The person's family history can be approached in a similar manner to their personal history by asking for information that relates to the problems or issues they have described. It is also appropriate to check whether any family members have any physical or mental health problems that might have a hereditary element such as breast cancer or psychosis.

Physical health

Assessment of physical health should consider the following areas:

- Does the person have any current physical health problems such as diabetes or heart disease?
- What is the state of their physical health, for example are they obese?
- Is their mental state impacting on their physical condition? Specific areas to check are appetite, sleep and libido.

- Use of intoxicants such as tobacco, alcohol or drugs.
- Where patients and service users are already being treated with medication, the nurse should check whether they are experiencing any side-effects that are having an adverse effect on their physical health. Some of the medications prescribed for psychosis (e.g. lithium carbonate, clozapine and olanzapine) have serious side-effects. Being able to assess and identify side-effects from medication is an important part of the nurse's role.

Assessment of physical health is covered in detail in Chapter 9.

Assessment of risk

One specific type of assessment that has increased in frequency over recent years is the area of risk assessment. Here, the purpose or goal is to assess to what degree the patient presents a risk of harming themselves or others, or to what degree they may be at risk of harm from other people. Risk assessment may also be part of a broader process known as the care programme approach (Warner 2005). This is a statutory framework for working with people with mental health problems. A recent report investigating the involvement of service users in risk assessment and management suggests that nurses should be working more actively to involve service users in the process (Langan & Lindow 2004).

Assessing risk involves finding out whether the patient has any previous history of risk behaviours, identifying current risk behaviours such as hearing voices urging the person to harm themselves or others (command hallucinations) and gathering information about their alcohol or drug use. The assessment of risk may require patients to discuss or disclose information about events that are upsetting, and it therefore requires nurses to be sensitive about how they manage this. Each practice environment will have a protocol for the assessment of risk, and you should make sure you are familiar with the content.

METHODS OF ASSESSMENT

The most common methods for structuring the process of assessment are the use of observation, questionnaires and rating scales, and interview (Ryrie & Norman 2004).

Observation

Observation is one of the essential skills and, as discussed in Chapter 2, this involves observing self, others and the environment. In this chapter, we will focus only on observation of others. In Chapter 2, we presented a model of descriptive observation that involves noticing appearance, behaviour and speech. Aspects of the person's appearance to notice include eye contact, facial expression, their body and grooming, including clothing. Behaviour is observable by noticing posture, movement, activity and interaction with others. Observation of speech involves paying attention to the process of speech, for example the speed and volume, as well as the content.

Questionnaires and rating scales

Questionnaires and rating scales are examples of formal assessment tools. Many different tools have been developed, and it is important to select the one relating to the area you want to assess. These tools can be administered by staff or can be completed by patients or service users, when they are known as 'self-rating tools'.

Your mentor or other member of staff will need to guide you through their use. We list some of the main tools below, and many of them are available to download from www.mentalhealthnurse.co.uk (go to 'Resources' and then 'Assessment tools'). Information about most of these tools can also be found in McEvoy (2003). You should be aware that some tools are bound by copyright law and must not be used without consent (see Box 7.2).

Global rating scales

Health of the Nation Outcome Scale (HoNOS) (see www.rcpsych.ac.uk/cru/honoscales/). This 12-item scale was developed to measure clinical

Activity box 7.2 **Assessment tools**

In order to familiarize yourself with assessment tools, next time you are in a practice environment, find out what assessment tools are being used.

Discuss how to use them (e.g. whether they are used by staff or given to patients to complete) with your mentor.

outcome in relation to behaviour, impairment, symptoms and social functioning.

Mental state/symptoms

Brief Psychiatric Rating Scale (BPRS; Overall & Gorham 1962). As its name indicates, this scale was developed to assess the presence of a range of psychiatric symptoms such as anxiety, depression and psychosis.

Beck Depression Inventory (BDI; Beck et al 1996). Once specific symptoms such as anxiety, depression or psychosis have been detected, it may be useful to focus on the symptom in more detail. The BDI is a self-rating tool that assesses the presence and severity of depression.

Side-effects scale

Liverpool University Neuroleptic Side Effect Rating Scale (LUNSERS; Day et al 1995). This is a self-rating tool that identifies the side-effects of neuroleptic medication.

Barnes Akathisia Rating Scale. This focuses specifically on the presence of akathisia (restlessness), a side-effect of neuroleptic medication.

Social functioning

Social Functioning Scale (Birchwood et al 1990). Social functioning can be impaired through illness, and it may be useful to assess formally how the person manages daily activities such as social relationships, budgeting, shopping and eating.

Interview

Interviewing is essentially an interpersonal process, and effective interviewing draws on the skills necessary for developing therapeutic relationships (Chapter 2), observation (Chapter 3) and communication skills (Chapter 6). A general goal is to elicit information in order to plan care. In many contexts, the interview format is prescribed, and the nurse is required to follow this structure. This is often the case in acute settings or when a patient first has contact with services, and there is a set of forms for the nurse to complete.

Preparation

Interview preparation has a number of components. Find out what information about the patient is already known, for example from case notes or in a referral letter. There are different views regarding whether to seek as much information as possible before the interview or whether to go in with an open mind and not be influenced by the opinion of others. Both views have their merits and their risks, and the decision may rest in part on what sort of assessment is being conducted. In the case of conducting a risk assessment, it is necessary to draw on as much existing information as possible. As well as consulting written sources, people can provide valuable information. This includes members of the health and social care team or family, friends and carers of the patient.

Managing time

Nurses need to give clear information to patients regarding the length of the interview, the type of information to be discussed and the potential outcome. Being clear about these areas is partly about respect for the other person's time, especially as patients have often taken additional time to travel to the appointment. It also increases the likelihood of being able to use the time effectively. The amount of time available is important as an interview of 15 minutes will cover different information from one lasting an hour. As long as everyone knows how much time they have, they can then decide what to bring in and what to leave out according to the time available.

Although the whole of the interview is important, the beginning and ending should be given particular attention as they are transition points. The interview occurs within a time boundary, so both parties have to shift their energy and attention from what they were doing before to focus on assessment. It is part of the nurse's role to help the patient manage this transition. By clarifying the length of the interview at the start of the meeting, the ending has already been indicated. It can be helpful to signal the ending by commenting when there are 5 or 10 minutes left. This can help to focus both parties' attention and provides an opportunity for any significant information that has not been mentioned to be raised at this point.

Managing content

Patients will not necessarily know what sort of information we would like them to give, unless of course we tell them. This is why it is important to give clear information at the beginning of the interview. Patients will also have their own expectations about the process, and it can be helpful to check these. For example, the patient may not have been given a clear explanation about why a referral has been made or may have misunderstood what they were told. They might have particular issues that they want to discuss that the nurse might not consider wholly relevant to the assessment process. If these expec-

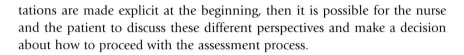

tations are made explicit at the beginning, then it is possible for the nurse and the patient to discuss these different perspectives and make a decision about how to proceed with the assessment process.

Communication skills

As a novice interviewer, it can seem rather daunting when you think about everything that happens during an interview, such as communicating effectively, managing time, using questioning skills, as well as taking notes and trying to remember and respond to what you have been told by the patient. It is important to be realistic and acknowledge that you will not be able to manage all these aspects at first but, with practice, you will develop your skills repertoire. Thinking about communication skills is a good way to begin (see Box 7.3).

Listening

Communication skills are often organized into two categories, verbal and non-verbal (Chapter 6). In the context of assessment, where the primary goal is to find out about the other person, listening is a key skill. We can demonstrate that we are listening by using both verbal and non-verbal behaviours.

Reflecting back

Reflecting back involves repeating back what we have heard the person say as far as possible using the same words they have used. This is often used for

Activity box 7.3 Communication skills

When you are on clinical placement, observe an assessment interview carried out by a colleague. Identify some of the communication skills you saw being used and think about why they were used. What was the nurse trying to convey to the patient? Were there any other communication skills that could have been used?

Ryrie I, Norman I (2004) Assessment and care planning. In: I Norman and I Ryrie (eds) *The Art and Science of Mental Health Nursing. A Textbook of Principles and Practice*. Maidenhead: Open University Press.

Warner L (2005) *Review of the Literature on the Care Programme Approach*. London: Sainsbury Centre for Mental Health.

www.mentalhealthnurse.co.uk (go to 'Resources' and then 'Assessment tools').

www.rcpsych.ac.uk/cru/honoscales/index.htm

8

Care delivery and interventions

I'm realizing how providing good mental health care is more than just thinking about people's mental state. It also involves being aware of the person's physical state as well as their social situation.

Second year student nurse

INTRODUCTION

Delivering care to patients and service users is at the heart of nursing. It incorporates a number of aspects, including communication, interpersonal relationships, assessment and health promotion (Nursing and Midwifery Council 2002). These are used to develop a plan of care with patients, service users and carers, which is then implemented and evaluated. There is an expectation that mental health practitioners should be able 'to deliver evidence-based interventions that facilitate recovery and meet the needs of mental health service users, their carers and families' [Sainsbury Centre for Mental Health (SCMH) 2000: 15].

In this chapter, we have used the framework of interventions presented in *The Capable Practitioner* (SCMH 2000). The interventions are organized into four categories: medical and physical care; psychological interventions; social and practical interventions; and mental health promotion. We briefly discuss each category and then focus in detail on one example. In order to illustrate how the interventions may be used in practice, a clinical scenario is developed in relation to each group of interventions, and we consider how the four essential skills (therapeutic relationship, observation, roles and reflection) relate to care delivery.

INTERVENTIONS

Mental health problems can have a significant impact on individuals and their families, especially if the problems persist. Multidisciplinary teams have developed in order to provide patients with a range of interventions.

As discussed in Chapter 1, the report *The Capable Practitioner* (SCMH 2000) identified the capabilities required to implement the *National Service Framework for Mental Health* (Department of Health 1999). *The Capable Practitioner* presents four groups of interventions based on biopsychosocial and health promotional models. These are:

- medical and physical health care
- psychological interventions
- social and practical interventions
- mental health promotion.

It is not expected that all practitioners will have expertise in every area; rather, that nurses should work with their managers to ensure that they are clear about the expectations of the post that they hold and what the service is required to deliver. For example, 'early signs monitoring' is one of the psychological interventions that a nurse in a community mental health team would be expected to deliver. However, a liaison nurse in an accident and emergency department would probably not deliver this intervention, but could be expected to have knowledge of other psychological interventions such as crisis intervention and resolution.

MEDICAL AND PHYSICAL CARE

This group of interventions includes physical care, physical treatments such as medication and the management of aggression, and covers the following areas of care (SCMH 2000):

- assessment of mental and physical health needs
- managing anger, violence and aggression
- participating in the delivery of electroconvulsive therapy and other physical treatments (see www.rcn.org.uk/mhz/good_practice/new_guidance_on_ect_21_apr_2005)
- ability to participate in arrangements to address the physical health needs of service users by appropriate joint working with primary care
- facilitating concordance with treatment.

Assessment of mental and physical health needs

People with schizophrenia and bipolar disorder have higher levels of physical ill health than those without mental health problems. The reasons for this are complex but include side-effects of neuroleptic medication (e.g. weight gain, diabetes and cardiac problems) as well as higher levels of lifestyle behaviours, such as smoking, that are associated with heart disease and strokes (www.drc-gb.org). Nurses are well placed to monitor patient's physical health and offer information on smoking cessation. See Chapter 9 for information on improving physical well-being.

Managing anger, violence and aggression

Although a detailed account of managing aggression is beyond the scope of this text, prevention of violence is always the first priority. The chapters on observation and reflection in the first section of the book will provide a useful base for developing your skills and understanding. Although profiles of patients more at risk of violence have been identified, staff attitudes and behaviours and the environment are also extremely important (Sookoo 2004). If violence does occur, it is essential that it is managed in a way that ensures the safety of all present. This is taught in specific courses (e.g. control and restraint sessions) that will be a mandatory part of your training.

Facilitating concordance with treatment

There are a number of terms currently being used to describe how patients and service users participate in treatment and receive interventions. The term 'compliance' is now considered to represent a paternalistic approach to care with an implicit expectation that patients will follow the doctor's orders. Adherence and concordance are preferred terms, as they reflect a more contemporary partnership approach to treatment and care. Concordance, in particular, implies agreement between the parties. However, at the time of writing, the word 'concordance' does not appear to be widely used in practice. We have used the term 'managing medication' based on the work of Grey and colleagues at the Institute of Psychiatry (Gray et al 2002).

Nurses are likely to be involved in the delivery of all the medical and physical health care interventions outlined above at some point during their training or career. Facilitating concordance with treatment relates to all aspects of treatment including psychological, social and medical or physical interventions but, here, we will focus on medication. Adherence to treatment is an important issue. It is clear that mental health practitioners can and have developed many physical and psychological treatments that have been proven to be effective. However, many treatments have also proved to be unacceptable to the people for whom they have been developed, and this contributes to non-compliance.

Investigations into 'non-compliance' with medication have shown that there are many reasons why patients do not take medication as prescribed. These include problems with side-effects as well as feeling better and therefore not seeing any need to continue with treatment. Interestingly, it has also become apparent that 'non-compliance' with medication is not confined to mental health, but is a general issue and includes patients prescribed a range of treatments such as antibiotics and those with chronic conditions such as diabetes. Compliance rates between patients with psychiatric conditions and those with physical disorders are relatively similar (Cramer & Rosenheck 1998).

Managing medication

In mental health, there has been a gradual move towards understanding health and illness by the use of models that incorporate a number of perspectives, for example the biopsychosocial model. This model acknowledges the importance of biology, psychology and social factors in contributing to who we are as individuals, our relative health and our potential for ill health. In accordance with this model, it is important that patients are offered a range of interventions, not just medication (National Institute for Clinical Excellence 2002).

Medication has long been an important treatment for a range of disorders such as psychosis, anxiety and depression. Currently, medication is at the heart of many treatment regimens, and nurses continue to have a key role in all aspects of medication management. In order to administer medication safely, the nurse needs to draw on biological knowledge that includes pharmacology, anatomy and physiology as well as psychological approaches to managing medication that include exploring the individual's beliefs about treatment.

Safety is of paramount importance when administering medication, and guidelines are available from the Nursing and Midwifery Council (2004). Most trusts will also have policies relating to the administration of medication, which nurses should consult. The ethical aspects of treatment are of equal importance, particularly as they relate to consent.

Goals of medication management

Whenever medication has been prescribed, the nurse will have the following specific goals:

- Administering medication. The nurse is most likely to be directly involved when the individual is an inpatient or during acute episodes when they are being seen at home by members of a home treatment team.
- Monitoring the effects and side-effects of medication. Nurses often have the most contact with patient and service users, and they are therefore best placed to observe for the effects and side-effects of medication. Neuroleptic medications have many side-effects including weight gain, effects on glucose levels, cardiac arrhythmias and Parkinsonian side-effects such as tremor and rigidity.
- Providing information about medication and the condition for which it has been prescribed. This includes identifying symptoms that might respond to medication and working in partnership with the patient to maximize adherence. For example, one patient might prefer taking a single dose of medication daily whereas another might find it easier to remember to take medication if they take a dose two or three times a day.

Medical and physical interventions and the essential skills

The essential skills can be seen as an important resource in the delivery of interventions. By having these skills in mind, it becomes more likely that the nurse will keep the patient as the main focus rather than the intervention. There are times, particularly when we are less experienced, when the 'task' or activity (e.g. administering medication) can become the goal at the expense of the therapeutic relationship. However, the essential skills can help us to stay 'on track' as we pay attention to the information drawn from observation as well as attending to the therapeutic relationship and identify what is the most useful role at any time. Reflecting on this later can also help us to learn more about what happened and explore whether we would act in the same way if a similar situation arose again (see Box 8.1).

Observation

As discussed in Chapter 2, this involves noticing self, others and the environment. Observation is often the first skill we use, as accurate and effective observation provides us with information about the patient's general condition as well as the effects and possible side-effects of interventions. Monitor-

Activity box 8.1 Managing medication

You are a student nurse working with a staff nurse in an acute admission ward and assisting with the administration of medication. Ahmed is a 28-year-old man who has been on the ward for 2 weeks. He has not come for his medication, so the staff nurse asks you to call him.

You find Ahmed sitting by himself in the dayroom and ask him to come for his medication. As you speak to him, he stands up and swears at you, says the medication is killing him and he won't take it and tells you to leave him alone.

Think about what you would **observe** in this situation, how you would develop a **therapeutic relationship**, which **role** you would need to adopt and how **reflection** might help you learn from this experience.

ing our own reactions may also help to provide information about what the other person is experiencing.

- What do you see when you enter the dayroom? What do you notice about Ahmed's appearance and behaviour?
  - How is he sitting, for example is he hunched over in his chair looking at the floor or sitting upright?
  - When he stands up, is his body passive or moving, for example does he gesticulate with his arms?
- What do you observe about the tone of Ahmed's comments?
  - Is his voice soft or loud?
  - Did he say anything about how he was feeling?
  - Do you think he sounded sad or perhaps despairing or maybe angry or even afraid?
- Notice your own reaction. If he sounds angry you might find yourself thinking 'How dare he speak to me like that, I'm only doing my job.' You might feel frightened by his anger and fear for your safety. Similarly, if you thought he was sad or in despair, you might feel sad or concerned that he might harm himself.

Therapeutic relationship

All aspects of delivering care and interventions are mediated through the relationship between the nurse and the patient. It is very easy for issues of power and control to become dominant in situations where patients are being asked to do something that they do not want to do. Therefore, it would be important to acknowledge Ahmed's point of view immediately. The nurse should aim to keep the lines of communication open. In order to do this, it is essential that Ahmed is offered an opportunity to discuss what he has said about the medication killing him. Some medications can have serious and potentially harmful side-effects, and the student should seek advice from the nurse administering the medication regarding how to assess this.

Ahmed has also said that he wants to be left alone, so the nurse should try to respond to this statement. You could say 'I know you want to be left alone now but could we discuss this later?' Allowing him to make a decision here could help him to feel that he has some control within the situation. It is possible that he may not agree to meet later. If so, you should discuss with the staff nurse whether to approach him again.

Role

The three core roles are delivering care, providing information and managing emotions. The situation (Box 8.1) sounds as though it was emotionally charged, for Ahmed and the student, and so managing emotion will be the priority. One way to approach this is to attend to the facts and the feelings that have been expressed. Acknowledge the fact that Ahmed has said he does not want to take his medication by paraphrasing what he has said. For example, you might say 'I know you don't want to take the medication. Can you tell me why you feel it's killing you?'

In addition, try to reflect the feelings he has expressed. In the scenario, Ahmed has not actually said how he is feeling, so you would have to use information drawn from observation to assess his emotional state. Sometimes, our own emotional reaction is triggered by the other person's emotional state. For example, if Ahmed is angry, you might feel angry that he has sworn at you. Similarly, if he seems very anxious or afraid, you may feel fearful about what he might do. Another common reaction is to feel upset and perhaps think that you must have done something wrong. You should try to contain how you feel until you can discuss this with a more experienced colleague. Try to be calm in your response to Ahmed. For example, you might say 'I'm sorry you feel so upset (or worried or angry), I'll let staff nurse know what you've said.'

The primary role was delivering care, in particular the administration of medication, so you need to address this by reporting to the staff nurse. You should also let Ahmed know that you will pass this information on. The staff nurse will need to decide what action to take, for example talking to Ahmed and assessing for side-effects. This could result in Ahmed's medication being changed. Your interaction with Ahmed, as well as the outcome, will also need to be documented.

Reflection

Reflection is largely concerned with evaluating the contact between patient and nurse. This changes from moment to moment, and reflection is a means for nurses to check whether they are managing themselves in a way that is useful to the patient. Another element of reflection is decision making, particularly deciding whether the interaction is effective or whether a change needs to be made. Reflection needs to occur both 'in action', that is while the nurse is with the patient, and also 'on action', that is following the contact (Schon 1987) (see Chapter 5). As a student, developing your skills of reflection will be a gradual process. Reflection-in-action begins by being aware of what you observed about yourself, the patient and the environment. You should also be aware of what role you are in and reflect on whether you need to change roles.

Reflection-in-action

In this scenario (Box 8.1), we noted that the student approached Ahmed in the role of delivering care and interventions, in particular administering medication. However, on making contact with Ahmed, i.e. by observing him, it became clear that the student needed to take up the role of managing emotions. In such a situation, the student will also have to make decisions about timing. This includes thinking about whether it is possible to interrupt the medication round and offer to spend time with Ahmed. It also means reflecting on whether this is the best time to discuss what has happened with Ahmed. If he is very angry, having some time to calm down may make it easier to discuss his feelings, whereas if the main emotion he is experiencing is fear, this might build up and become harder for him to manage if he has to wait. The student will also have to decide whether they have the knowledge and skills to discuss this with him or whether it would be better for Ahmed to be seen by a more experienced colleague.

Reflection-on-action

Reflection-on-action will follow the same process of reviewing what you observed and what roles you took up, as well as reflecting on what decisions were made and the eventual outcome. The key difference is that this can be done without the pressure of being in the situation.

When reflecting on a situation such as the scenario in Box 8.1, you should start by remembering what happened in as much detail as possible. This includes thinking about what you observed about yourself and the other person, as well as identifying any assumptions you might have made. So consider how you approached Ahmed and how you responded as the situation unfolded. If you were completely surprised at his reaction, think about whether there were any clues to his mood that you might have missed. Go back to what you noticed when you first entered the dayroom. Consider the fact that Ahmed had not come for his medication and what you thought that meant at the time (for example, that he had forgotten or was doing something else). When reflecting on such a situation, remember how you approached the patient and the first words you spoke. For example, did you ask him to come for his medication, did you say hello and ask him how he was, or did you say that you had been looking for him? There is no right way of approaching this situation but, by reflecting, you become aware of the way in which different approaches may impact on what follows. Finally, reflect on whether you would behave in the same way if such a situation happened again or whether there is anything you would do differently (see Box 8.2).

Activity box 8.2 **Reflection-on-action**

Look again at the examples of medical and physical health care interventions on p. 149.

Think back to your placement experience and identify a situation that relates to one of the headings (e.g. managing anger, violence and aggression).

Briefly review what happened by considering each of the four essential skills (therapeutic relationship, observation, roles and reflection), as we did for the scenario with Ahmed.

PSYCHOLOGICAL INTERVENTIONS

Mental health nurses need to be able to participate in the delivery of evidence-based psychological interventions. At present, cognitive behavioural interventions form a significant part of the evidence base, which is why they are included in the list below. *What Works for Whom? A Critical Review of Psychotherapy Research* (Roth & Fonagy 2005) discusses a range of different psychological interventions, and the National Institute for Health and Clinical Excellence (NICE, formerly the National Institute for Clinical Excellence) has produced guidelines on the management of a number of conditions including schizophrenia, depression and anxiety, eating disorders and post-traumatic stress disorder. It is important to visit the NICE website regularly (www.nice.org.uk) to ensure you have the most up-to-date recommendations.

Evidence-based psychological interventions include the following:

- early intervention, early signs monitoring, relapse prevention
- psychoeducation
- crisis intervention and resolution
- cognitive behavioural interventions
- psychotherapeutic and other talking treatments

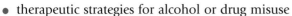

- therapeutic strategies for alcohol or drug misuse
- cognitive and behavioural family interventions.

Psychoeducation

Interventions may be aimed at both individuals and their family. Although the term 'psychoeducation' is not that well defined, it originated as an intervention for the families of people with schizophrenia. It became apparent that some family members were misattributing signs of illness to personal qualities, and this was having a negative impact on how they related to the person. For example, lack of motivation is interpreted as laziness rather than seen as a symptom of illness. People who are diagnosed with a mental illness may also not fully understand how the illness affects them. Consequently, psychoeducation may be offered to individuals and their families to help them understand the impact of illness.

Psychotherapeutic and other talking treatments

There are a number of influential psychological models including cognitive behavioural therapy (CBT), psychoanalytic, psychodynamic and systemic models. All place an emphasis on both the therapeutic alliance and the use of specific techniques to bring about change.

Therapeutic strategies for drug and alcohol use

Some of the psychological interventions listed above are aimed at people with particular problems such as alcohol and drug use. The approaches include a detailed assessment of the problem and the use of techniques such as motivational interviewing. The aim is to change (substance-using) behaviour, but it is recognized that this is a slow process that can happen in stages. Motivational interviewing works specifically with the person's desire (or motivation) to change at each stage.

Other interventions are designed to be used at specific time points such as during times of crisis (crisis intervention and resolution) or when someone first becomes unwell (early intervention). In order to illustrate how the core skills are applied to psychological interventions, we will use early signs monitoring as an example.

Early intervention, early signs monitoring and relapse prevention

Although these interventions have been grouped together, there are key differences that will be outlined briefly before focusing in more detail on 'early signs monitoring'. The terms will be discussed as they relate to working with people experiencing psychosis.

Psychosis

Psychosis is a medical term used to describe a group of disorders in which there is a change in the person's ability to process information and recognize reality. People may experience hallucinations and hold strong beliefs that are not shared by others (delusions), as well as having extreme mood changes. Concentration is commonly affected by these experiences, which can make it difficult to follow conversation and communicate with people (British Psychological Society 2000). Psychosis is often used as shorthand for a range of conditions including schizophrenia and bipolar affective disorders. In both the literature and clinical practice, it is also increasingly being used to include the experiences described above (i.e. hallucinations and delusions), regardless of whether a formal diagnosis has been made. Used in this way, it is considered to be less stigmatizing than diagnostic terms, particularly schizophrenia.

Early intervention

Early intervention is used to describe care that is focused on the early phase of psychotic illness. There has been a gradual recognition that the care needed at this time point is different from that required by people who have been ill for a number of years. It includes early detection of illness as well as improving engagement between individuals (and their families) and services in order to help people access appropriate treatment and support (McGorry 2004).

Relapse prevention

The term 'relapse prevention' was initially used in the field of substance misuse, but the term has also been applied to people with a history of psychosis. A number of studies have investigated how relapse may be reduced by interventions such as early signs monitoring, compliance therapy as well as family interventions and cognitive behavioural interventions (Gleeson 2004).

Early signs monitoring

Early signs monitoring is one of a number of psychosocial interventions for people experiencing psychosis (see Box 8.3, overleaf). It can be used with those who have already had a number of relapses, as each relapse increases

> ### Box 8.3 Early signs monitoring
>
> Ahmed has been discharged from hospital and referred back to the community mental health team. While he was in hospital, his medication was reviewed; he is now taking a different antipsychotic and is experiencing fewer side-effects. He has now had six admissions in 7 years, and the team has suggested a course of psychological interventions.
>
> Through discussions with Ben, his community psychiatric nurse (CPN), Ahmed describes how he and his sister came to the UK from Somalia when they were teenagers to escape from the civil war in which their parents were killed. When he started college, he began to hear voices telling him he should have died. He thought he was possessed by djinn (evil spirits). He still hears these voices.
>
> Ahmed believes the spirits caused him to become unwell, and he is worried that he may end up back in hospital. Ben discusses early signs monitoring with Ahmed, and he agrees to work with Ben.

the likelihood of having another one. The work involves three stages, has a number of elements and usually takes place over a period of time rather than in a single session (Birchwood et al 2000).

Stage 1   Agreement to work on preventing relapse

In order to participate in this work, the patient needs to believe that it is possible they might have another relapse. The nurse should talk to the patient to establish the patient's understanding of what has happened to them. For example, they may believe they have a mental illness or that they have been affected by stress or that their neighbours have tried to harm them. It is not necessary for people to believe they have a mental illness in order to participate in this work. However, if someone were strongly convinced that they would never find themselves in the same situation again, they would probably not see any reason for undertaking this work.

Stage 2   Identify signs of relapse

This involves gathering information from the individual and others including family, friends and other professionals regarding previous relapses to identify the sequence of events. The patient needs to consent to information being sought from others. The nurse should explain that the person's family and others may have noticed changes in their behaviour, on their own or with others, which the individual may not be aware of. In this way, a more complex picture of the period before relapse can be developed.

Personal relapse signature

The nurse should ask the patient to recall what they noticed in the weeks or days leading up to the most recent relapse and identify their feelings, behaviour and thoughts as well as any physical changes. The aim is to build up a detailed picture that is known as a personal relapse signature.

Stage 3   Development of a relapse drill

The information from the personal relapse signature is used to develop a plan or relapse drill, which should include detailed information about how to respond to the different relapse signs. The action plan (see Box 8.4) should include a range of strategies, such as exercise or relaxation techniques, that the person can implement themselves or do with the help of family and friends, but should also make it clear when professional advice should be sought. Ahmed should have a copy of the plan to refer to, and a copy should be kept in his notes.

SOCIAL AND PRACTICAL INTERVENTIONS

In order to attain and maintain good mental health, we all need access to housing, health care, work, education and leisure as well as good personal and social networks. Having a mental illness is distressing and difficult enough, but it can also have a major impact on people's quality of life. Illness may disrupt schooling and education as well as leading to long periods of sick leave or unemployment, which can in turn make it more difficult to gain further employment. Mental illness also impacts on families,

---

Box 8.4 Example of an action plan for Ahmed

Relapse signs	Action
Feeling irritable	Talk to my sister, tell her how I feel
Starting to worry that something terrible is going to happen	Contact CPN on . . .
Not sleeping at night	Have a bath before going to bed Take extra medication at night

for example parents may take on a carer role for an adult child with a mental health problem. In contrast, some children provide care for parents with mental health problems and find their childhood is curtailed. It is important, therefore, that assessment is comprehensive and takes account of the individual and the social context in which people live. Treating mental illness is only one part of helping people to improve their mental health (see Box 8.5).

Therapeutic relationship

Ben will have spent time developing a good therapeutic relationship with Ahmed that has allowed trust to develop. Within the relationship, Ahmed has identified some areas that are of concern to him: his loneliness and worries about getting on with people. He has also identified some goals for the future related to developing IT skills and improving his English. Ben now needs to decide how best to help Ahmed with these issues.

 Activity box 8.5 Roles and social and practical interventions

Ahmed continues to meet Ben, his CPN, regularly. Over time, Ahmed describes feeling lonely and isolated. He sees his sister often and occasionally goes to a café where he meets other Somali men. He is worried that, if they find out he has been in hospital, they won't have anything to do with him. Consequently, his visits to the café are infrequent.

Ahmed also starts to talk about his plans for the future. He would like to develop his IT skills and improve his English, but doesn't know how to do this. He's also worried that if he goes to college, he won't get on with the other students.

Think about the different roles Ben might use (see Chapter 4) to help Ahmed to deal with some of the issues he is worried about.

Ben and Ahmed decide that improving his skills is the first step. There is also the possibility that he might meet some new people on a course. They agree that the course would also help to boost his confidence, and that this might make it easier when he meets Somali men in the café.

Providing information

After discussion with Ahmed, Ben may decide to take on the role of providing information. This might involve finding about courses on Ahmed's behalf or finding some preliminary information, such as telephone numbers and email addresses, and letting Ahmed acquire the information himself. Ben will need to know not only whether Ahmed wishes to do this himself, but also whether he has the ability and resources to do so. For example, Ahmed may be very familiar with using a computer but not know how to enrol on a course.

Managing emotion

If Ahmed decides to enrol for a course at a local college, he may feel quite apprehensive. Helping Ahmed to manage his emotions at this point will be very important. This might involve normalizing how he is feeling as well as helping him to prepare for college. Ben could discuss Ahmed's previous experiences of education with Ahmed and explore what he felt he managed well, as well as any areas of difficulty. Ben might offer Ahmed additional support when he first starts at college, such as more frequent meetings or contact by telephone. Ben would also assess Ahmed's mental state during this time to monitor how he was managing the additional stress.

MENTAL HEALTH PROMOTION

The Sainsbury Centre for Mental Health (2000) organize the capabilities for mental health promotion into two groups. The first is providing information to individuals so that they can use it to improve their mental health, thereby reducing the incidence of illness. The second is about addressing issues of discrimination and exclusion at a broader level, including organizations and communities. As a student nurse, you will probably have more involvement with the former, but you also need to develop awareness about how to approach mental health promotion at a more systemic level, which includes:

- understanding the continuum of mental health promotion and prevention
- awareness of the impact of mental health on physical health

Activity box 8.6 Mental health promotion

Think back to the scenarios about Ahmed (Boxes 8.1 and 8.3).

Try to identify some issues relating to mental health promotion that might be appropriate for Ahmed.

• working with individuals and organizations to facilitate self-help, strengthen social networks and reduce discrimination and social exclusion (see Box 8.6).

Illness to well-being

You will probably have noticed that the scenarios reflect a shift in emphasis for Ahmed from illness to well-being. When he was an inpatient, managing his illness was the priority. This continued to be important when he returned home, and a key role for the nurse is delivering care as well as maintaining and developing a therapeutic relationship. As the acute phase of illness subsides, it becomes possible to focus on improving his mental health.

If successful, the social and practical interventions outlined above will contribute to improving Ahmed's mental health. The development of the relationship between Ben and Ahmed will also be significant. It is possible that their contact will reduce over time as Ahmed develops his own resources. This might include developing an increased range of coping skills, leading to more confidence in his abilities. Increasingly, patient or service user groups and organizations are also offering support and resources to each other.

Mental health promotion

Finally, it is important to consider the broader issues of mental health promotion that are implicit within the scenarios. People with mental health problems are commonly excluded from employment and training (Office of the Deputy Prime Minister 2004), and this social exclusion can exacerbate mental health problems. In addition, people from ethnic minorities and young men are at even greater risk of exclusion.

As a student, you should try to think about the patients and service users you work with in relation to their community and local facilities. Just because facilities such as colleges, libraries and leisure centres are available locally, it does not necessarily mean that everyone will be able to access them. Try to develop your own knowledge about local resources and assessing whether people are able to access them.

SUMMARY

- Nurses deliver care through a range of interventions that include medical and physical care, psychological, social and practical interventions, as well as mental health promotion.
- Medical and physical care includes assessment of mental and physical illness as well as facilitating adherence to treatment.
- Evidence-based psychological interventions include medication management and cognitive behavioural therapy for psychosis.
- Social and practical interventions can have a significant impact on quality of life.
- Mental health promotion should be addressed at both an individual level and a community and social level.
- The four essential mental health nursing skills (therapeutic relationships, observation, taking on different roles and reflection) need to be considered whenever care is being delivered.

References

Birchwood M, Spencer E, McGovern D (2000) Schizophrenia: early warning signs. *Advances in Psychiatric Treatment* 6, 93–101.

British Psychological Society (2000) *Recent Advances in Understanding Mental Illness and Psychotic Experiences.* Leicester: BPS.

Cramer JA, Rosenheck R (1998) Compliance with medication for mental and physical disorders. *Psychiatric Services* 49, 196–201.

Department of Health (1999) *National Service Framework for Mental Health.* London: Department of Health.

Gleeson JFM (2004) The first psychotic relapse: understanding the risks and the opportunities for prevention. In: JFM Gleeson and PD McGorry (eds) *Psychological Interventions in Early Psychosis. A Treatment Handbook.* Chichester: John Wiley and Sons.

Gray R, Wykes T, Gournay K (2002) From compliance to concordance: a review of the literature on interventions to enhance compliance with antipsychotic medication. *Journal of Psychiatric and Mental Health Nursing* 9, 277–284.

McGorry PD (2004) An overview of the background and scope for psychological interventions in early psychosis. In: JFM Gleeson and PD McGorry (eds) *Psychological Interventions in Early Psychosis. A Treatment Handbook.* Chichester: John Wiley and Sons.

National Institute for Clinical Excellence (2002) *Clinical Guidelines. Core Interventions in the Treatment and Management of Schizophrenia in Primary and Secondary Care.* London: NICE.

Nursing and Midwifery Council (2002) *Requirements for Pre-registration Nursing Programmes.* London: NMC.

Nursing and Midwifery Council (2004) *Guidelines for the Administration of Medicines.* London: NMC.

Office of the Deputy Prime Minister (2004) *Mental Health and Social Exclusion. Social Exclusion Unit Report.* London: ODPM.

Roth A, Fonagy P (2005) *What Works for Whom? A Critical Review of Psychotherapy Research*, 2nd edn. New York: Guilford Press.

Sainsbury Centre for Mental Health (2000) *The Capable Practitioner. A Framework and List of the Practitioner Capabilities required to Implement the National Service Framework for Mental Health.* London: SCMH.

Schon D (1987) *Educating the Reflective Practitioner.* San Francisco: Jossey-Bass.

Sookoo S (2004) Therapeutic management of aggression and violence. In: I Norman and I Ryrie (eds) *The Art and Science of Mental Health Nursing. A Textbook of Principles and Practice.* Maidenhead: Open University Press.

www.drc-gb.org

www.nice.org.uk

www.rcn.org.uk/mhz/good_practice/new_guidance_on_ect_21_apr_2005

9

Improving physical well-being

> *I was shocked when I realized how little I had thought about physical well-being. At times the signs of poor physical health were clear but I wasn't really seeing what was there. Now I really try to pay attention to this aspect and I think it makes a difference to how people feel.*
>
> Community mental health nurse

INTRODUCTION

There is growing evidence that the physical health of people with mental health problems is poor compared with that of the general population, and they have a reduced life expectancy (Seymour 2003). Yet people with mental health problems are frequently seen by a range of health professionals, including nurses, which suggests that the physical aspect of health has been overlooked by professionals.

The majority of people with mental health problems are seen in primary care; a small percentage are referred to specialist mental health services, and only a small proportion of these are admitted to hospital (Goldberg & Huxley 1992). However, many people being seen by mental health services will also be in regular contact with their general practitioners (GPs). This may result in both primary and secondary care services assuming that the other is responsible for a particular aspect of care such as physical health, when in fact neither is taking responsibility.

Within mental health services, the key structure for assessing the needs of people with mental health problems and reviewing care is the care programme approach (CPA) (see p. 207), and physical health should be included as part of this assessment. However, the increased morbidity and mortality rates for people with mental health problems suggest that, even if physical health needs are being identified, they do not appear to be being addressed.

Recent research has investigated the views and experiences of service users in relation to physical health care. Repeatedly, this is showing that health professionals are underestimating the importance of this to patients and service users (Dean et al 2001, Edwards 2005). As the *Chief Nursing Officer's Review of Mental Health Nursing* in England (Department of Health 2006a) notes, nurses are well placed to assess and address physical health needs.

This chapter discusses the concepts of health and well-being. Although the emphasis here is on physical well-being, this is a slightly artificial separation as many of the factors that are important to physical health also affect mental health. The main physical health problems experienced by mental health patients and service users are identified. The main causes of physical health problems associated with mental ill health are social exclusion, lifestyle factors such as smoking, the physical effects of illness and the side-effects of medication. These are discussed in order to help nurses to understand the complex nature of the problems relating to physical ill health. We discuss assessment methods, including observation, which, in relation to physical health, includes clinical observations such as temperature recording as well as the use of questionnaires and rating scales. The topic of health promotion

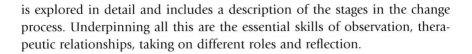

is explored in detail and includes a description of the stages in the change process. Underpinning all this are the essential skills of observation, therapeutic relationships, taking on different roles and reflection.

HEALTH

The traditional way of thinking about health is as the absence of disease. However, this definition has increasingly been seen as too narrow as it focuses on the presence or absence of a medical condition, and as too negative as it does not encompass any positive aspects of health. In order to address these concerns, the World Health Organization (WHO) stated in 1948 that health is 'a state of complete physical, mental and social well being' (World Health Organization 1948). This definition has also been criticized because it suggests that there is a kind of gold standard for health that people can aspire to, but few will attain.

The WHO later revised its definition to include an individual's ability, on the one hand, to realize aspirations and satisfy needs and, on the other hand, to adapt to a changing environment (World Health Organization 1984). This more dynamic understanding emphasizes that health depends on an individual's personal characteristics, the ability to achieve aspirations and to adapt to changing circumstances, rather than on objective measurement. This means that 'health' has different meanings for people depending on their abilities and circumstances; a person with a physical disability has different criteria for health from a professional athlete, for example. Similarly, an elderly person may have an understanding of health that includes living with one or more chronic conditions such as arthritis. From this perspective, health is related to quality of life, rather than to disease or disability. This way of thinking about health involves all aspects of a person's life. Quality of life depends on well-being that is not only physical and mental, but also emotional and spiritual. It also includes many social factors including environmental circumstances, such as housing, and economic factors, such as employment and income.

PHYSICAL HEALTH

The number of research studies into the physical health and well-being of people with mental health problems has increased over the last decade. The literature broadly covers two areas: investigations into levels of morbidity and mortality; and interventions aimed at improving physical well-being.

The life expectancy of a person diagnosed with schizophrenia is reduced by 10 years compared with someone who does not have a mental health problem (Brown et al 2000). A diagnosis of schizophrenia or bipolar disorder increases the risk for physical disorders such as coronary heart disease, diabetes and respiratory diseases (Phelan et al 2001). Depression and alcohol use are also associated with increased rates of physical disease.

Health and well-being are influenced by a range of factors that relate to individual and familial factors such as genetic inheritance, as well as social factors. There are a number of reasons why people with mental health problems may have poor physical health (Seymour 2003). These are:

- impact of social exclusion
- lifestyle factors
- physical effects of mental illness
- side-effects of medication.

Impact of social exclusion

Social exclusion is a term used to describe what happens to groups of people who are disadvantaged as a result of discrimination, and is associated with unemployment, poor housing, ill health and family breakdown. Many people are affected by social exclusion, including people with mental health problems. The impact of social exclusion is far reaching and affects the individual's ability to access work and training or education as well as health care (Office of the Deputy Prime Minister 2004). It also impacts on people's social support networks, which are often eroded over time. Social exclusion and poverty go hand in hand, so people with mental health problems commonly live in poor housing. It is ironic that, although people are no longer incarcerated for long periods as in the days of the asylum era, social exclusion has resulted in many people with mental health problems remaining as cut off from their community as if they were still segregated in a hospital even though they live in the community.

Social exclusion is fuelled by stigma and discrimination. Judi Chamberlain (a consultant in survivor perspectives) notes that 'stigma' locates the problem in the individual, whereas 'discrimination' 'puts the onus where it belongs, on the individuals and groups that are practicing it' (Sayce 2000: 15). The impact of social exclusion is a reduced quality of life as people either are deliberately excluded from or feel unable to access services and facilities that others take for granted. This includes access to health care. The evidence suggests that people with mental health problems do not receive the physical health care that a person without a mental health problem would expect from health professionals and, in this respect, they are experiencing discrimination. Many people will also have internalized a more generalized form of discrimination that shapes their image of themselves. For some, this means that their dominant identity is being a patient. This can lead them to see themselves as being very different from people who do not have a mental health problem. Seymour (2003) reports that those mental health service users who knew that health promotion material was available in GP surgeries thought that it was not relevant to them because of their mental health problems.

Lifestyle factors

Health and well-being (both physical and mental) are associated with a number of factors including our own behaviour. The term 'lifestyle factors' is used to refer to behaviours of our own that can impact on health (Box 9.1).

Behaviours can have a negative or positive effect or a mixture of both. Here, we will focus on factors that have a negative impact on health. The key lifestyle factors that contribute to poor physical health are smoking, poor diet and lack of exercise. Drugs and alcohol also impact on health and are discussed under 'Physical effects of mental illness'.

Smoking

Adults with a range of mental health problems including schizophrenia and depression are more likely to smoke than those without a mental health problem (McNeill 2001). Even higher rates of smoking are associated with being in hospital (Cormac et al 2005). Seymour (2003) describes a 'smoking culture on psychiatric wards' where smoking becomes a way to pass the time

 Activity box 9.1 Lifestyle behaviours

Think about your own physical health. Identify any behaviours that you think may have a positive or negative effect on your own physical health and well-being.

and people reported smoking more than usual when they were in hospital. Smoking contributes to cardiovascular, respiratory and circulatory disorders.

Diet

A poor diet in people with mental health problems can lead to obesity, although medication is also considered to be a contributory factor (see p. 174). The diet of people with mental health problems has received much less attention than that given to smoking. However, there is some evidence that people with schizophrenia have diets that are high in fat and low in fibre and some vitamins, and this is associated with disorders of the cardiovascular and gastrointestinal systems (McCreadie et al 1998). Poor nutrition, especially in relation to B vitamins, has long been associated with excessive alcohol use.

Exercise

Another lifestyle factor associated with obesity (which is part of a national problem) is low levels of exercise. Sedentary lifestyles increase the risk of developing diabetes, high blood pressure and heart disease (Richardson et al 2005). Taking regular exercise confers not only physical benefits but has also been shown to have an impact on depression and some anxiety disorders (O'Connor et al 2000, Lawlor & Hopker 2001). Despite this, exercise is rarely included as part of treatment regimens.

Criticisms of 'lifestyle' factors

There is a risk that, by focusing on individual behaviours that affect health, the individual is seen as being responsible or is at risk of being blamed for any health problems that develop. The term 'lifestyle' implies a freedom to choose or reject a behaviour, whereas the reality is much more complex. Smoking, for example, is an addiction so, for many people, it is not as simple as just deciding to stop.

The effects of illness may also have an impact, for example anxiety is a core component not only of anxiety disorders such as phobias but is commonly present in psychotic illnesses including schizophrenia. Social anxiety is characterized by a fear of negative evaluation by others and can impact on people's willingness and ability to engage with other people. For some, this results in leading quite a solitary life and being reluctant to go out. This could then contribute to a more sedentary lifestyle.

In practice, many people, especially those who experience social exclusion, may feel they have few choices about how they live. They may also not have access to relevant information that could help them to make informed choices. They may also lack the skills and resources to make changes, or may not recognize opportunities for change when they arise. Because of this, they may feel they have little control over their own health. Therefore, it is important to see the lifestyle aspects as one of a number of factors that may be contributing to poor physical health.

Physical effects of mental illness

Having a mental illness can affect people's ability to maintain good physical health and well-being in a number of ways. The effect may be direct, most notably in relation to addictions. All addictive substances, for example alcohol or heroin (and nicotine), affect the brain and have a mood altering effect. In addition, these substances also have an effect on other parts of the body, which can result in significant physical damage. For example, alcohol has a toxic effect, particularly if it is consumed over many years or in large quantities. Alcohol affects many parts of the digestive system including the liver, stomach and pancreas as well as affecting heart muscle.

With drugs that are taken through smoking, such as cannabis or heroin, the main effect will be on the respiratory system, although other systems are also affected. Some drugs such as heroin can also be injected, and this brings the risk of infection through blood-borne agents, for example hepatitis C and the human immunodeficiency virus (HIV).

Having a mental illness also has the potential to affect the immune system, leading people to be more susceptible to developing infection. There are various explanations for this including that it is due to the chronic effects of anxiety and trauma that leave the body in a constant state of physiological arousal (the flight or fight response). Low self-esteem is another factor that is associated with mental illness and may affect the ability of the immune system to deal with infection.

Side-effects of medication

The main groups of medication prescribed for mental health problems are:

- antipsychotics (used for positive symptoms of psychosis such as hallucinations and delusions)
- antidepressants
- mood stabilizers (used to treat mood disorders)
- anxiolytics (to treat anxiety).

All medications have side-effects, but this section will focus on antipsychotic medication as this group has a greater impact on physical health.

Antipsychotic medication

Antipsychotic medication was introduced in the 1950s; it blocks dopamine receptors in the brain. It is this blocking action that produces both the desired effect on symptoms and the unwanted or side-effects. Antipsychotics (also known as neuroleptics) such as chlorpromazine, haloperidol and flupenthixol have been used for many years. They have many side-effects including extrapyramidal symptoms (EPS), also known as Parkinsonian side-effects as they mimic the symptoms of Parkinson's disease. These side-effects include tremor and rigidity.

The so-called 'atypical antipsychotics' have been developed more recently and tend to have fewer extrapyramidal side-effects. However, although all antipsychotic medication is associated with weight gain, the atypical antipsychotics, especially olanzapine and clozapine, seem to be more likely to cause this than the older medications. As noted above, obesity contributes to a range of physical disorders such as hypertension and cardiovascular disease. The rates of impaired glucose tolerance and diabetes seem to have increased since the introduction of the atypical neuroleptics (Taylor et al 2005). Again, clozapine and olanzapine are particularly associated with this effect.

Some side-effects, although rare, are so serious that regular monitoring is a condition of their use. An example of this is agranulocytosis which can be caused by clozapine. This is an acute condition where there is a dangerous reduction in the number of white blood cells.

Many side-effects are not as potentially harmful as those described above, but they can nonetheless have a serious effect on quality of life. For example, drowsiness can be a side-effect of antipsychotics and antidepressants. Blurred version can interfere with reading and watching television, while constipation can cause physical discomfort. As a student, it is important that you become familiar with the possible side-effects that patients may experience in order to be able recognize and respond to the presence of side-effects.

ASSESSMENT

As discussed in Chapter 7, the most common methods of assessment are by observation, interview and the use of questionnaires and rating scales. Each method will produce different types of information, which can help to build up a more complex understanding of the individual's perspective and circumstances as well as their needs.

Observation

Observation is one of the four essential skills (see Chapter 3) that can provide nurses with crucial information about a patient or service user's physical well-being as well as their mental state. Some aspects of an individual's physical state will be immediately apparent as soon as we see them, such as whether they are under- or overweight, whereas others such as blood pressure will only be known through measurement. Through observation, we can learn much about the other person by paying attention to their appearance (Box 9.2).

In relation to physical health, you need to develop a sense of what is normal or usual for people who are in good physical health. This will help you to develop your ability to recognize when you are observing something that is not within the normal range. For example, a person who is in good physical health would not usually have a blue tinge to their skin.

In order to be aware of appearance, you will use information drawn from four of your senses: sight, hearing, touch and smell (Figure 9.1).

Sight

You may learn a lot about someone's physical state by paying attention to what you see when you are with them.

Physique

You should start with a general sense of how the person looks and then look more closely at particular aspects of their appearance. Notice whether their body size matches their physique or if they seem clearly over- or underweight.

> **Activity box 9.2 Observation of appearance**
>
> Think about someone you met recently who you thought was physically unwell.
>
> What did you notice about them that made you think they were unwell?

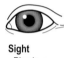

Sight
- Physique
- Skin
- Movement
- Posture

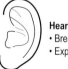

Hearing
- Breathing
- Expressions of pain

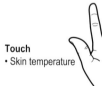

Touch
- Skin temperature

Smell
- Bodily fluids e.g. urine
- Intoxicants e.g. tobacco

Figure 9.1 Observation of physical appearance.

Skin

Notice skin colour, e.g. does the person appear pale or flushed, or does their skin have a yellow or blue tinge? Skin tone – does the skin look very dry or dehydrated or are there signs of sweating? Is the skin intact or are there signs of injury such as cuts, bruising or swelling? Are there signs of needle marks and, if so, are they clean or do they look infected?

Movement

Can the person move their limbs freely or are there signs of tremor or rigidity? Notice whether there are signs of movement being limited in any of the limbs.

Posture

Observe the person's posture and how they hold their body. Sometimes, when a person experiences pain in the chest or abdomen, they may hold or protect that area when they cough or move.

Other

Other effects (that may result from side-effects of medication or other causes) that can be seen include hypersalivation, drowsiness, hypotension, e.g. dizziness on standing up.

Hearing

Information about someone's physical state can also be gathered from paying attention to what you hear.

Breathing

Notice whether there are any signs that the person is having difficulty breathing, such as wheezing, shortness of breath or coughing.

Expressions of pain

An example of this is wincing or a sharp intake of breath that may be heard when someone experiences pain or discomfort.

Touch

Physical contact may come in the form of a handshake when meeting someone. If you notice that the person looks unduly hot or cold, you may wish to feel their forehead or hand in order to feel their skin temperature. You should seek the person's verbal agreement before you make physical contact.

Smell

If the person does have a strong smell, it is likely that you will notice this. You should try to identify the source of the smell, for example whether it is body odour, urine or faeces. It is also possible to smell intoxicants such as alcohol, cannabis or tobacco, although this does not necessarily mean the person has been using them. Nonetheless, you should try to develop an ability to detect whether what you can smell is on the person's clothing or being excreted on their breath or through their skin.

Clinical observations

These are clinical observations that are used to measure the individual's physical condition. These observations can be taken to provide information about the person's current state and also to establish a baseline for future comparison. In an inpatient setting, there will be guidelines regarding what clinical observations should be taken routinely, and you should familiarize yourself with these. Usually, a full set of observations is taken and recorded on admission.

The Maudsley Prescribing Guidelines (Taylor et al 2005) recommend that patients taking antipsychotic medication should have their blood pressure monitored, especially during the early stages of prescribing or when they are changed to a new medication. They also recommend that weight be monitored. A recent publication by the Department of Health has recognized the role that nurses can play in improving physical health and recommends that patients should have an annual review of blood pressure, pulse, body mass index, blood tests and urinalysis (Department of Health 2006b).

they are still present at the next meeting. Other symptoms should be referred to a doctor for assessment.

Screening checks

If any checks are overdue, you should discuss this with the patient or service user. There may be many reasons why appointments have not been made, including anxiety about the procedure, forgetting to make an appointment or not being registered with a surgery. For some people, raising the issue will be enough to make an appointment, but some people will need assistance in order to do this.

INTERVENTIONS

On p. 170, we described the four factors (social exclusion, lifestyle, physical effects of mental illness and side-effects of medication) that contribute to poor physical health in people with mental health problems. Each of these factors needs to be considered when designing and delivering interventions to improve physical well-being.

Social exclusion

In the UK, social exclusion has been recognized as a significant issue, and the government has set up a dedicated unit to address the issues (Office of the Deputy Prime Minister 2004). As a student, you should be aware of how social exclusion affects the patients and service users that you meet. If social exclusion is the problem, then broadly speaking social inclusion is the solution. Burns (2004: 19) describes social inclusion as 'deinstitutionalization's second phase' and argues that it is not enough simply to move patients out of hospital and into the community.

We may use resources for many reasons, such as education and training (e.g. colleges and libraries), health and recreation (e.g. swimming pools and parks) and leisure (e.g. cinema). As a student, it is important to talk to patients and service users and find out about which local facilities they use. By doing this, you will begin to get information about how connected they are with their local community. It will also help if you know or find out about what facilities are available locally so that you can offer this information if requested (see Box 9.3).

In the past, facilities such as gyms and a range of groups were often provided through mental health services. It has been argued that this perpetuated some aspects of social exclusion by keeping people with mental health prob-

Activity box 9.3 Community resources

Think about the local area or community where you live or work.

List all the community resources you use and think about why you use them.

lems out of 'mainstream services'. Increasingly, service user networks are becoming an important provider of user-led facilities that access local facilities such as cinema. They offer support to access facilities through a group or befriending service and also provide opportunities for people to take on different roles in the organization. As a student, you should aim to find out about local service user networks.

Lifestyle factors

There has been limited research into healthy living interventions for people with schizophrenia, although the most effective studies targeted smoking cessation (Bradshaw et al 2005). Physical exercise has been shown to have a beneficial effect on depression as well as having the potential to improve physical health and well-being (Lawlor & Hopker 2001). Nurses rarely seem to have been involved in planning or delivering these interventions. However, this is gradually changing (Ohlsen et al 2005, Department of Health 2006a).

Behaviours that contribute to improving physical health (lifestyle factors) are addressed in detail under health promotion on p. 190.

Physical effects of mental illness

Some physical health problems are associated with the use of addictive substances, and it is therefore important that the person is offered treatment for their addiction. They will also require medical assessment and treatment for any physical conditions such as hypertension or respiratory disorders. Some of the physical problems may be irreversible and will need ongoing monitoring by a medical practitioner. Nurses who are in regular contact with patients and service users are also well placed to assess their physical condition and encourage medical referral if there are signs of any deterioration.

Side-effects of medication

We noted earlier that the side-effects of many medications can impact on physical health as well as being unpleasant for the person who is experiencing the side-effect. Nurses therefore need to be familiar with the side-effects of medications.

Awareness of the presence of side-effects may come from the patient, through observation of the patient or through assessment or measurement. Many patients learn to recognize the presence of side-effects and may indeed self-manage them through medication or other means. The presence of side-effects can be particularly distressing for people when they are first being treated, which is why low doses are recommended when first prescribed. However, side-effects can still arise, and the patient may come to staff with an awareness that something is happening without necessarily knowing what is causing it (see Box 9.4).

At other times, patients may not be aware that they are experiencing side-effects, and so it is important for nurses to observe and to be alert to the

Activity box 9.4 Identifying side-effects of medication

Think of a patient you met recently during a placement and remember what medication they were prescribed.

What are the main side-effects of this medication? Where can you find this information?

How would you know if the patient was experiencing these side-effects?

possibility of side-effects. A useful tool for the assessment of side-effects is the Liverpool University Side Effect Rating Scale (LUNSERS) (Day et al 1995). This is a simple self-rating scale that patients and service users can use themselves to detect the presence and severity of side-effects. Because of the frequency of side-effects, nurses usually become adept at deciding which side-effects require an urgent response. However, all side-effects should be taken seriously and, if you think the person is experiencing side-effects, you should report this to a registered nurse.

PROMOTING PHYSICAL HEALTH

Health promotion is a term that refers to a number of interventions aimed at helping people to acquire the knowledge, skills and knowhow to make informed choices about their own health. The WHO reflects this by defining health promotion as 'the process of enabling people to increase control over, and to improve, their health' (World Health Organization 1986). This process involves providing people with information that will help them to make informed health decisions, and facilitating people to adapt their lifestyle by learning new skills and integrating new ways of living into their lives.

The emphasis is on helping the patient or service user to take responsibility for their own physical health, rather than having an intervention imposed on them by a nurse or family member. We all have experience of being nagged about something, whether it is tidying our room, doing our homework or losing some weight, and the effect is to make us feel irritated and resentful about it. We may eventually perform the task, but our motivation is to avoid the nagging, rather than because we appreciate the benefits of having a tidy room, etc. The aim of health promotion is to enlist the person's own desire for better health in making positive changes to their lifestyle to help in achieving this. This does not mean leaving them to get on with it but, in the context of a therapeutic relationship (see Chapter 2), helping them to think about their health and to work out what behaviour changes they could realistically make, helping them get started and providing support and encouragement.

For some people, the benefits of apparently 'unhealthy' behaviour may be more important than the risks. Despite being exposed to up-to-date and easily understandable information about the risks, they may choose to continue the behaviour. This is their informed choice and should be respected. There may be other health behaviour that it is easier for them to change at the moment, and they may later be able to contemplate more adventurous changes.

A model of the change process is provided here followed by an outline of the process of assessing a person's health promotion needs and planning for making changes. Some issues in the implementation of changes are then discussed, including the key lifestyle factors affecting mental health service users, and strategies for making and maintaining changes. The nurse's information-giving role is then described. Finally, some notes on the evaluation of lifestyle changes are included.

Stages in the change process

Prochaska and DiClemente (1982) have suggested that people pass through a number of stages in identifying, deciding upon and making changes to their health behaviour. This process is characterized as a cycle as there are often several attempts at making a change before a new behaviour is successfully adopted, for example a smoker may try to give up several times before being successful.

As Figure 9.2 shows, there are five main stages to the cycle, but there is also a preliminary (precontemplation) stage, which prefigures a person's entry into the change process, and another stage (exit), which marks a person's successful change in their behaviour and exit from the change process cycle.

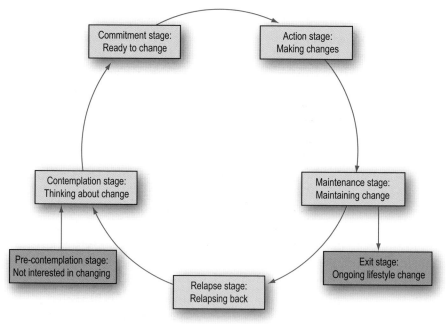

Figure 9.2 Stages of behaviour change (adapted from Ewles & Simnett 2003).

Precontemplation stage

This is the state that precedes any wish to make behavioural changes. The person carries on their usual lifestyle and may be unaware of any health risks associated with their behaviour, or have only a limited understanding of their consequences. Alternatively, the person may have some awareness of the risks but believes that these are outweighed by the benefits. At this stage, they may be accessible to health education material that provides them with accurate and easily understood information abut the risks so that their choice of whether to carry on with that behaviour is well informed.

Contemplation stage

This is the entry point into the process of change where the person has an awareness of a need for change and has begun to contemplate the possibility. At this stage, information about different options might be helpful, for example someone contemplating giving up cigarettes might find information about different ways of managing withdrawal symptoms (such as nicotine chewing gum and nicotine patches) useful, as well as information about local smoking cessation programmes and groups. They may also need help and guidance with making decisions about which risk behaviours to focus on, for example it may be unrealistic for a man who is a heavy smoker and over-weight with a sedentary lifestyle to take up an exercise programme, stop smoking and go on a reducing diet all at the same time.

Commitment stage

At this stage, the person makes a definite decision to make a change to their behaviour. Here, they may need help with formulating a plan that is SMART (specific; measurable; achievable: realistic; time oriented) as well as with planning for situations of temptation and episodes of relapse. For example, a young woman who is trying to lose some weight and usually has a chocolate croissant with her friends during her coffee break at work will need to plan how she is going to manage her coffee breaks without having a chocolate croissant. With planning, she may manage to avoid the coffee break problem but find herself craving chocolate by lunchtime and, one day, give in to the craving. Does this mean she has failed and should abandon her diet?

Action stage

This is the stage at which the person begins to implement the change they have been planning for. It may be useful at this stage to provide a support structure for the person in the form of a support group of other people making a similar change, such as a weight loss group or an exercise group. This provides both peer pressure for the person to succeed and a support structure they can turn to for boosts in motivation. Alternatively, they may find this is better provided in an individual session focusing on their progress and coping strategies.

Maintenance stage

This stage stretches beyond the initial motivation of making the change into the longer term of trying to form the new behaviour into a new habit. At this stage, the person has overcome the initial resistance and has gone for some time without their previous behaviour. They may feel they have conquered it and be vulnerable to sudden cravings, or they may become demoralized and suffer losses of motivation. For smokers, for example, this can occur between 3 and 6 months after their last cigarette as they begin to move away from a 'one day at a time' approach to a more 'never again' perspective. This is a critical period as, on one hand, the person is close to success and, on the other, they are very vulnerable to relapse. In this stage, it may be helpful to emphasize the positive benefits of the behaviour change. This needs to be done in terms that they value. For example, a woman who has been struggling to lose weight may appreciate being able to wear more flattering clothes, or a young man who has been struggling to cut down his alcohol consumption may appreciate being able to run around on a football field. It may be helpful to plan strategies for managing temptation with the person; these may include distracting themselves with thoughts of something else, or perhaps telephoning the nurse or a trusted friend for encouragement and support. From the maintenance stage, a person may either successfully exit from the change process or relapse and continue in the cycle.

Exit stage

The exit stage occurs when the person has successfully incorporated a new behaviour into their lifestyle. There is no predictable point for this as it will vary from person to person – some people will be free from the habit very quickly, whereas others may experience temptations or cravings for several years. People tend to revert to habitual patterns at times of stress, so old broken habits may reappear temporarily from time to time, but they are usually easily overcome and, unless they persist, they need not be regarded as relapses.

Relapse stage

Most attempts to change behaviour are likely to suffer a relapse at some point. This may be short lived, and the person may be able to reassert their commitment and re-enter the action and maintenance stages with relative ease. But, for other people, the relapse may be more catastrophic, leaving them feeling hopeless and defeated. At such times, the help that is called for is encouragement and positive reinforcement of their achievements. It may also be useful to try and re-engage the person with their commitment to change by emphasizing the benefits. The relapse stage leads back to the contemplation stage, where the person begins to think again about the possibility of making a change. At this point, it is important to evaluate carefully the factors and circumstances that led to the relapse and incorporate them into the plan.

Assessment of health promotion needs

Like any other nursing intervention, health promotion should be carefully planned and targeted to an identified aim. The starting point is to conduct an assessment of the person's current lifestyle and their understanding of its relationship to their health. This can be included as part of the physical health assessment (see p. 178).

The assessment of health promotion needs focuses on the person's current health behaviours and their knowledge about the associated risks, as well as their attitude to making changes to these behaviours and potential barriers to change. The assessment aims to identify which of their behaviours may have a negative impact on their physical health and how prepared they are to contemplate changing these. This information can help you to work out how you may usefully intervene to help them make the changes. In order to do this, it is useful to position the person on the change process cycle for each of their behaviours. For example, see Box 9.5 (overleaf).

Planning

The change cycle will clarify the person's readiness to contemplate or implement changes to different behaviours and start to make plans. Although the plan may stipulate some direct interventions from the nurse, for example providing health education information about a specific issue, it will mainly focus on changes to be made by the service user. The nurse's main roles at this stage are to support the person's motivation for change and to facilitate the planning process. To do this, the nurse needs to use their communication skills (see Chapter 6) to listen closely to the patient and to help them clarify their priorities and formulate SMART objectives and goals (see Chapter 10). The nurse also provides experience and knowledge about different interventions that may help the person to make and maintain changes, such as a shopping and cooking group to help with changes to eating habits. As well as identifying the change to be made, the action plan should include resources the person can use for support and strategies for coping with temptation. For example, see Box 9.6.

Box 9.5 Assessment of John's health promotion needs

John is a 28-year-old unemployed single man. His habit is to rise late and spend most of his time watching television. When he was younger, John was very fit and played football for the local amateur team. More recently, he has taken up smoking and has become overweight. He would like to regain some of his fitness and, to this end, has recently tried to control his 'comfort eating'.

In relation to his diet, John is in the action stage, as he is aware of the problem and has begun to take action. John is less aware that his inactivity is also a problem, although he is hoping to start playing football again at some stage. He is therefore in the contemplation stage for his inactivity. It has not yet occurred to John that smoking is also having a negative effect on his health and is likely to interfere with his hopes of getting fit again. For this, he is still in the precontemplation stage.

See also Boxes 9.6, 9.7 and 9.8.

Box 9.6 Helping John with planning

John has already identified that he aims to regain some of his former fitness and that, to do this, he needs to lose some weight and, at some stage, do some exercise. The role of his nurse Mary at the planning stage, in addition to providing support and positive reinforcement, is to help John translate these aims into plans. He may need help to formulate his ideas into specific, realistic and achievable objectives, which are time oriented and can be measured (SMART), and shorter term manageable goals. Mary can also help John to plan how he will go about achieving his goals and objectives (see 'Interventions') and anticipate some of the difficulties he might face and help him to plan how to cope with these. The plan may also outline what Mary will do to support John as well as to inform him about the effects of his smoking.

Implementation

Different strategies to make and support change may be adopted depending on the lifestyle change that is required. Nurses can provide assistance with identifying useful strategies and support in maintaining change. They also have a specific role in providing accurate and up-to-date information. For example, see Box 9.7.

Box 9.7 Helping John to implement his plan

John has already identified that he aims to regain some of his former fitness and that, to do this, he needs to lose some weight and, at some stage, do some exercise. The role of Mary, his nurse, is to help him to formulate these into SMART objectives and goals and to plan how he will go about achieving these.

In relation to his weight, John is in the action stage of the change process as he has already begun to try and cut down. Mary will help him to clarify his target weight and the timescale for achieving this. She may also suggest he keeps a diary of everything he eats and drinks so they can review it together and monitor the nutritional balance of his diet. This may highlight John's understanding of his diet. Perhaps he has cut out biscuits and cakes, for example, but continues to drink several bottles of carbonated sugary drinks each day. Mary will be able to educate John about balanced nutrition by providing him with information and helping him to make sense of it. Mary may be aware of other resources John could use to help him lose weight. For example, there may be a local weight loss group he could join where he would meet others with similar difficulties and gain support and positive feedback. However, this may not appeal to John, and Mary will need to listen carefully to him to understand the specific support he is likely to find helpful.

In relation to his inactivity, John is in the contemplation stage as he is aware that, at some point, he will need to take action, but he has not yet clearly identified what the action will be or how he will go about it. Mary's role is to help John to move into the action stage. It may help John to get started if Mary can give him a better understanding of the health effects of inactivity, particularly when associated with excess weight. She may also help him to establish a plan by clarifying how fit he would like to become and what activities will help him to

---

achieve it. John's wish may be to join the local amateur football club, but he may need to gain a basic level of fitness beforehand to avoid becoming demoralized. Mary may be able to help him formulate a suitable basic exercise regime, or he may need more specialized help such as a fitness instructor, a local gym or a circuit training group. It may also be useful for John to keep an exercise diary so that any practical or motivational problems can be easily identified.

In relation to his smoking, John is in the precontemplation stage, as he has not yet begun to contemplate any change. In the short term, Mary may be able to provide him with health educational material, such as leaflets, and be prepared to explain or discuss these with him so he has a better understanding of how his smoking is likely to impair his attempts to improve his fitness. In the longer term, if he starts to contemplate a change in his habit, she will help him to plan whether he wants to cut down or stop altogether and whether to use nicotine patches or chewing gum or neither to manage the withdrawal symptoms. She may also know of a smoking cessation group he could join.

Key lifestyle factors

For mental health service users, the key lifestyle factors that contribute to poor physical health are smoking, poor diet and lack of exercise. Alcohol and drug use are also important, and all these factors may be compounded by lack of occupation. There are specific issues associated with each of these factors that affect which health promotion strategies and lifestyle changes are appropriate:

Smoking

Although a person may acknowledge that smoking is an undesirable behaviour that has a negative effect on their physical health, they may not be able to contemplate stopping altogether in the short term. However, even reducing the number of cigarettes they smoke each day can have a benefit for their health. Achieving a reduction in their consumption may encourage them to stop altogether at a later date.

Mental health service users report smoking more heavily during periods of inpatient care, and Seymour (2003) describes a smoking culture on psychiatric wards where smoking becomes a way to pass the time. This suggests that there may be changes that can be made to the inpatient environment and routine that would help to support reductions in smoking. These may include making it more difficult to smoke by restricting smoking areas. An important change would be to encourage inpatients to participate in useful and stimulating activity and replace a culture of inactivity with one of engagement and occupation.

There may also be organized smoking cessation groups in the area that can be accessed to provide information and support for people interested in changing their smoking habits. Alternatively, it may be possible to start a group if several service users and members of staff are interested.

Drug and alcohol use

It may also be difficult for a service user to contemplate cutting out an established drug or alcohol habit, although, as with smoking, reductions in consumption can still have beneficial effects. Another important aspect of health promotion with someone who continues to use drugs may be to help them to minimize the risks, for example helping injecting drug users to access clean needles and safely dispose of used ones. Where a person has a longstanding problem with their drug or alcohol use, it is advisable to seek guidance and support from specialist agencies.

Diet

There is a close link between food and emotional state; some people tend to overeat when they feel low. Reduced appetite and weight loss are also associated with depression, and people in a manic phase are likely to experience appetite disruption. Poor nutrition is a key feature of eating disorders such as anorexia and bulimia nervosa. People with mental health problems may be particularly vulnerable to some of the effects of poor diet, such as obesity, due to the side-effects of medication.

Changes in diet may be aimed at improving the nutritional value of the person's diet or at stabilizing their body weight or both of these and, as with smoking, even small changes can have beneficial effects on physical health. Changes need to be realistic and manageable for the individual as the main aim is for them to adopt and maintain a nutritionally balanced diet. The most useful changes are often reducing the intake of sugar, salt and fat.

Exercise

Physical exercise has been shown to have a beneficial effect on depression as well as having the potential to improve physical health and well-being (Lawlor & Hopker 2001). However, it may not be possible or desirable for a person to contemplate undertaking a vigorous exercise programme. Beneficial health effects can be achieved by small increases in activity, such as taking a short walk to the shops each day, walking to the next bus stop before catching the bus and climbing to the first landing before taking the lift.

Exercise needs to be graded to suit the person's ability. They should start gently and progress as their level of fitness improves. Gyms survive on the subscriptions of well-intentioned people who were unable to maintain the enthusiasm. An exercise programme is most likely to succeed if it can be integrated into the person's current lifestyle without too much difficulty.

Exercise can often be a rewarding group activity. People may enjoy playing low-level competitive sports, such as badminton, or team sports, such as five-a-side football. This can help to maintain their motivation as well improve communication skills and help develop friendships.

Occupation

Although inactivity, apathy and poor motivation are recognized 'negative symptoms' of some mental health problems, this can become a vicious cycle for some service users who have no way of occupying themselves which interests and engages them. Their apathy and boredom may be compounded by inactivity, and they may compensate with increased smoking, drug and alcohol consumption and overeating. This may reinforce a sense of power-lessness in relation to their health. Engaging with a stimulating activity can increase a person's sense of meaning and self-esteem.

Work is an important aspect of a person's identity that helps to establish and maintain their sense of their position and value in the community. For someone who has experienced mental health problems, it can be an impor-tant link to their responsible and competent 'not-patient' selves. Maintaining the connection with work can be crucial to a person's recovery, allowing them to rehabilitate and re-establish their role and self-respect. On the other hand, some people may find it difficult to cope with the demands of their previous work. Such people, along with others who were previously unemployed, may need help and support to find suitable employment. Guidance on preparing a CV and interview practice may be all that is required, while others may benefit from work experience programmes or assistance in accessing suitable training programmes.

For some people, it may not be possible to maintain the focus required to work because of temporary or more chronic problems with their concentra-tion and attention. However, they may be able to engage in stimulating and focused activities for shorter periods of time. These can be provided as inpa-tient groups or in specialist mental health services in the community, such as drop-in or day centres. Alternatively, they may access mainstream activity groups and clubs in the wider community. Any activity that stimulates and interests the person is valuable, but groups that focus on other aspects of their health behaviour may help them contemplate or implement additional life-style alterations. Useful activities may be shopping and cooking groups, diet groups or exercise clubs. Other activities might include discussions, for example about current affairs, or hobbies such as gardening or collecting.

Strategies for making and maintaining change

Making changes to possibly longstanding and habitual behaviours is difficult and demanding and needs to be supported by a range of strategies. These are designed to reinforce motivation at times of vulnerability and to focus on achievements and successes. People respond to different strategies depending on their attitude to the change they are making (see Box 9.5) and on their personality. A person who is highly motivated to change, with a good understanding of the health benefits, may be able to alter their behaviour with little support, whereas another person may have difficulty coping with the losses associated with the behaviour change and need more help to manage their motivation and to focus on the benefits.

Ewles and Simnett (2003) suggest some strategies for changing behaviour and coping with the temptation to relapse, which can be used by the person themselves with support from the nurse.

Self-monitoring

This involves the person keeping a detailed diary of the particular behaviour and their reaction to it. This helps them to see patterns that trigger particular behaviours and acts as a baseline from which they can measure success. For example, keeping a detailed diary of everything the person eats during the day may help them to see that they regularly have chocolate in the afternoon when they feel low. This will help them plan to manage the low period and avoid craving chocolate. The diary may also help the person to look back and see that, although they may feel a failure today because they succumbed to the chocolate in the afternoon, last week they also had chocolate in the morning and today is the only day this week when they have had chocolate. Ewles and Simnett (2003) suggest the diary should address such questions as:

- How frequently does the behaviour occur?
- The context it occurs in: what is happening for the person and around them?
- What event leads up to the behaviour?
- What happens afterwards and how do they feel?

Identifying costs, benefits and rewards

The losses or costs associated with making lifestyle changes can be difficult to bear and can undermine a person's motivation and resolve. For this reason, it is often helpful to be very clear about the benefits they are trying to gain by making the change so that they can remind themselves of these at moments of weakness. Some benefits of a change in diet, for example, may be weight loss and a renewed sense of attractiveness. On the other hand, these may take some time to achieve and, in the meantime, the person is missing the enjoyment of their previous habitual behaviour. It may be helpful to build smaller scale rewards into the intervening period to help reinforce success.

Groups

One way of helping to support lifestyle changes is for individuals to join together in groups. One advantage is that finite resources, such as a physical exercise instructor, can be available to a number of people at the same time. For some people, there are real benefits to this approach:

- Participants have the opportunity to discuss their lifestyle and health issues with other people in similar circumstances.
- Health information and knowledge can be shared and discussed, helping to consolidate understanding.
- Peer group pressure helps to support the individual's efforts.
- Group members can support each other at difficult times.

Some other people may find a group approach undermines rather than supports their efforts.

Finding a substitute

The person may be able to distract their attention from the behaviour change by replacing the undesired behaviour with something else. For example, chewing gum instead of smoking a cigarette or replacing a chocolate bar with an apple.

Changing associations

Sometimes, it may be important to change routines and habits that are associated with the undesired behaviour. For example, if drinking coffee during a work break has been associated with having a cigarette, it may help to drink tea or a cold drink instead. Similarly, if seeing a particular group of friends is associated with consuming alcohol, it may be helpful to see those friends individually or in a different context that is not associated with alcohol.

Rehearsing difficult situations

It may be useful for the person to anticipate situations when they are likely to be tempted to revert to the undesired behaviour and rehearse different ways of managing these. For example, they may practise refusing an offer of a cigarette or a drink, or plan a different route round the supermarket to avoid the cake stand. This will help them to manage situations that suddenly occur and may simply trigger the undesired habitual behaviour. They will be armed with an alternative response that can be used instead.

One day at a time

The prospect of never being able to indulge in a habitual behaviour again may be too overwhelming to contemplate, but the prospect of one day without it is more tolerable. This strategy can help with managing the initial stages of a lifestyle change when the temptation to revert to the previous behaviour is strong. By reducing the timescale to an hour, or even 5 minutes, it can also help to manage episodes of acute craving or relapse risk.

Providing information

Providing information is a key role for the nurse (see Chapter 4) and is an essential component of health promotion. The nurse acts as source of up-to-date and accurate information about health and lifestyle factors. This may mean searching out ready-made resources, such as leaflets or posters, to help the service users understand the issues. Alternatively, if few materials are available, it may be helpful for the nurse to investigate the subject and produce their own health promotional material. There may also be commercially available resources such as magazine or journal articles, DVD or CD-ROM packages. It is important that the nurse helps to interpret these materials to ensure that the service user gains an accurate understanding. This means both translating jargon into layman's terms and explaining sometimes complicated concepts in ways that convey their meaning but can be easily understood by the service user. This is a particularly important role for the nurse when discussing information obtained from the Internet that is not always accurate or up to date.

Evaluation

Evaluation of the change process can both help to monitor the progress of the changes that have been adopted and identify the helpfulness of support strategies on one hand and, on the other, provide useful material for post-relapse planning. For example, see Box 9.8 (overleaf).

If self-monitoring is used (see p. 193), the person will be able to see the progress of their behaviour change on a regular basis. For example, a person

> ### Box 9.8 Evaluating John's progress
>
> John and Mary, his nurse, may agree to meet weekly initially to discuss his progress. These meetings would focus on helping John to maintain his current plans by reviewing both his food diary and his exercise diary and identifying and analysing any problems he has had in the last week in maintaining his regime. They would discuss the circumstances and context of the problem and establish strategies to help him manage any similar problems over the coming week. These weekly meetings also provide an opportunity for John to gain some positive feedback and support on his achievements.
>
> They may agree to use one of these meetings each month to conduct a more detailed evaluation of John's progress. At these monthly meetings, they would revisit the assessment of his health promotion needs to clarify whether his needs had changed and what interventions had been helpful. Mary would then help John to develop new plans suitable to the revised assessment.

who is keeping a diary of their exercise can easily tell whether they have achieved their target. Similarly, a person who keeps a record of their weight can see at a glance whether they have gained or lost. This information is useful in short-term planning because it helps to identify whether the strategies are effective. If a person does not succeed in reaching their goals, they may become demoralized and vulnerable to relapse. This close monitoring of progress can therefore be useful, and it is important to identify the reasons for failure and make changes. The goal may be unrealistic and need to be adjusted, or there may be short-term crises that interfere with progress. Perhaps more short-term rewards are needed or strategies for managing fluctuations in motivation throughout the day.

Occasional relapses are to be expected as lifestyle changes are difficult to establish and maintain. However, it is important to carefully review the relapse and understand how it occurred. Somehow, the strategies adopted failed to provide the necessary support at the crucial moment. It is important to try and anticipate this situation in future and plan a strategy to manage it and prevent a future relapse.

It is also useful to review successful changes. This may provide useful information about which strategies the individual finds helpful in making changes, and this may be useful in planning future lifestyle changes.

10

Managing care

Managing care is not just about your own work with patients. You have to think about who else is involved, making sure everyone's up to date with the latest plans and decisions.

Third year student nurse

INTRODUCTION

As a student nurse, your early experiences during training will tend to focus on delivering care through direct contact with patients and service users. A registered nurse will supervise your work when you are a student, and part of what you will learn is how to manage yourself in order to deliver effective care. For example, you may learn how to use your time effectively by deciding between different priorities.

Decisions about managing care will be made by nursing teams and in multidisciplinary meetings, and the information that comes from your contact with the patient will contribute to the decision-making process. You will be expected to let staff know what you have observed and, as decisions are made and care plans change, information must be documented and communicated to all those involved in delivering care.

This chapter identifies three forums for managing care: individual, team and delegation. We also explore how systems such as the nursing process and theoretical models can be used to inform how care is managed. Although decisions about the management of care occur at specific points, such as care programme approach (CPA) meetings or ward rounds, monitoring the efficacy of care is ongoing. The essential skills of observation (Chapter 3) and reflection (Chapter 5) are especially useful for providing a method (observation) and a feedback loop (reflection) that can assist with this.

CONTEXTS FOR MANAGING CARE

The context is the setting in which care is managed. As noted in Chapter 4, each context will have its own goals, and different roles and accompanying behaviours can be used to achieve the goals. For the purposes of this chapter, we identify three different contexts for managing care (Figure 10.1):

- Individual. In this context, this refers to situations in which you are on your own with a patient. The primary responsibility is to report what happened to your mentor or nurse in charge.
- Team. This is the context in which most discussions regarding the planning and evaluation of care and interventions take place. Your key role here is to contribute relevant information to the team responsible for managing care.
- Delegation. As you become more experienced, you will be expected to delegate care to more junior students. Knowing how to do this effectively is an important part of managing care.

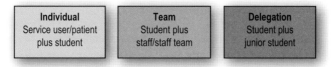

Figure 10.1 Contexts for managing care.

The individual context

The Nursing and Midwifery Council (2002) states clearly that, when you are a student, you are not accountable for your actions; accountability rests with the registered practitioner. There are nonetheless expectations regarding how you conduct yourself as a student when you have contact with patients, particularly if no other member of staff is present.

As a nurse, you will have to develop the ability to engage with and be present with the patient, but also train part of yourself to observe what is happening. If you think of this as paying attention to what is happening as it happens, you will probably find that you are already doing this. So, for example, you might be talking to an inpatient called Anthonia who tells you about her recent separation from her husband and suddenly starts crying. You might be aware that you think 'What do I do now?'

There are many different types of verbal responses you could make (see p. 119 – Heron's six-category interventions). However, in relation to managing care when you are on your own with a patient, there are only a limited number of general options available. These are:

- to continue what you are doing
- to stop what you are doing
- to do something different.

In the example above, you might check with Anthonia if she would like to continue speaking about her husband. Alternatively, she may wish to take a break to recover her composure (stop what you are doing), or it may be better to change to a less distressing subject (do something different). In all situations, you should report what happened to a registered nurse (see Box 10.1, overleaf).

Managing patient meetings

As a student, you will be expected to spend time with patients and service users through informal and planned contact. Some key principles can be identified to help manage this contact including introductions, endings and timing.

Activity box 10.1 Managing the individual context

Think of some situations in which you were alone with a patient when something happened that made you wonder what you should do next.

Looking back on how you managed, did you continue what you were already doing, stop what you were doing or do something different?

Introductions

Introductions are especially important when you meet someone for the first time. You must ensure that you identify yourself as a student nurse as well as by name (Nursing and Midwifery Council 2002). You may offer to shake hands if this seems appropriate to the context. You should try and present a calm, warm and friendly demeanour, speak slowly and clearly and pay attention to your own non-verbal behaviour (see Chapter 6).

Timing

The factors to consider here are the amount of time each participant has available for the meeting. It is important that patients are involved in determining the length of the meeting as this helps to build a collaborative style of working. It also reflects the fact that they too have lives in which they may have other commitments, and they may have a view on how long they would like the meeting to last.

The time and length of the meeting may also be affected by the person's mental state. For example, it is common for concentration to be impaired when unwell, and one way to try and manage this is to have several short meetings, perhaps of 15 or 20 minutes, rather than a longer meeting of 1 hour. The time of day may also make a difference, for example some people who are depressed find that their mood improves slightly during the course of the day, so would be able to participate more fully in a meeting during the afternoon (or evening if they are an inpatient) than one scheduled for the morning.

Environment

Mental health nurses now work in a range of settings including clinics, prisons, courts and schools as well as wards and people's homes. It is not uncommon to meet service users in public spaces such as a café or park. The physical environment is likely to influence what can be discussed. However, the impact of the setting will be affected by personal preferences. For example, some patients may prefer to discuss sensitive or personal issues in a park or open space rather than in a mental health setting, whereas others will prefer the privacy of an office.

In the nurse's own work setting, for example a ward or mental health centre, the nurse should prepare the environment before the patient arrives. When seeing someone at home, the nurse should assess the environment, taking into consideration factors that might intrude on the session. This might include noise from televisions or music systems. Family pets also need to be considered; if kept in the room, they may provide interruptions, but excluding them can also be problematic (for example, a dog barking outside the room).

Content

The content of the meeting will be partly determined by the amount of time available for the meeting. Ideally, the content should be agreed between the patient and the nurse. The care plan should contain information to guide the content of sessions. In addition, there are key time points that may influence the content. For example, during a final meeting, new material would not normally be introduced at this stage, and time would be spent acknowledging the ending of the relationship.

To summarize, there are a number of factors to consider when setting up a meeting. Some of these will be known before the meeting actually takes place, for example whether the patient and the nurse have met before. Other factors, such as what the home environment will be like when making a first visit, will be unknown. Nonetheless, the nurse has to develop a sufficiently flexible style of working to be able to manage this uncertainty.

Managing time

The ability to manage time effectively is an important skill in both a personal and a professional capacity. When you work with patients on your own, you will have to pay attention to how you manage time. This includes being able to negotiate and set times as well as keeping to the time limits that have been set. Repeatedly being late gives the person you are meeting the impression that you and your timetable are more important than they are. There is an inherent power imbalance between patients and nurses, and it is important to be aware that poor time management easily adds to the power differential (see Chapter 2). It is not always easy to master managing time as there are many pressures on time, and it is easy to find plausible reasons for being late. You could monitor your ability to manage time in different settings such as your placement, the university and in your personal life. If you become aware that this is something you find difficult, you should discuss it with your mentor or tutor.

The team context

Although the majority of care is actually delivered on an individual basis, much of the management of care is organized through teamwork (see Box 10.2).

If you produced a list of all the staff who contribute to the patient's care and well-being, it would probably be quite a long list. In order to be able to make sense of this list, you would probably start to group some staff together. For example, you might see that there are nursing teams, ward teams, multi-disciplinary teams as well as those providing support services such as cleaning, portering and ward clerks.

You would notice that most of the professions are from health and social care such as nursing, occupational therapy, social work, psychiatry and psychology. Staff from other services, for example the criminal justice system or education, may also be part of the team providing care. Other groups of staff include professionally non-affiliated support workers. Some staff such as nurses will always be part of the team, whereas others such as dieticians and physiotherapists may be called in on an occasional basis because of their input to a particular patient.

 Activity box 10.2 The staff team

Think about a ward or community setting where you have worked. Make a list of all the people who were part of the staff team.

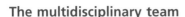

The multidisciplinary team

Multidisciplinary team working is highly complex, with many communications between different groups of professionals using different theoretical models to structure their work. By the nature of their close relationships with patients and service users, nurses often have a pivotal role in managing communication between the different groups of staff involved in care and facilitating their understanding of each other (see Chapter 6, Communication).

In this context, the main goal is for the team members to be able to communicate information they have regarding the patient or service user to each other (Onyett 2004). Managing the transfer of information from one person, team or service to another may appear quite simple, but can be difficult to achieve in practice. During the latter part of the twentieth century, a number of inquiries into serious incidents relating to patients have identified poor communication between services as contributing to the eventual outcome (see the Ritchie report 1994).

Different teams structure their work in different ways according to the client group they are working with, the setting they work in and the principles and priorities of their service. For example, teams working in community settings clearly have to be organized in different ways from those in inpatient settings. Also, changing thinking about the role of patients or service users in determining and managing their own care has called for more flexible ways of working. Recently, there has been a move away from services organized according to geographical location (for example, the 'South' community mental health team) to functional teams set up to deliver a particular service such as acute care, home treatment or early intervention (Burns 2004).

Care programme approach (CPA)

Many users of mental health services have complex needs requiring help with areas such as housing, finance, employment, education and physical health. No single discipline or agency can provide the variety of support that is often called for. The care programme approach, or CPA, is a statutory framework that provides a structure to help different disciplines and agencies work together effectively to provide co-ordinated care.

It has four main elements (Department of Health 1999):

- Assessment: a systematic and comprehensive assessment of the health and social care needs of the service user is carried out.
- Care planning: a plan is established clarifying how the identified needs will be addressed, and clearly indicating the roles of the different professionals and agencies.

- Care co-ordinator: a care co-ordinator is appointed who keeps in close contact with the service user and co-ordinates the other professionals and agencies in playing their part in the care (see below).
- Review: all interested parties (service user and carers, professionals and agencies involved) are involved in regular reviews of the health and social care needs of the service user and the progress of the care plan. Where necessary, changes to the care plan are agreed.

Care co-ordinator

Each patient has an identified care co-ordinator who is frequently a nurse (although it can be any professional involved with the patient's care). They are responsible for managing and co-ordinating the patient's care. The assessment and evaluation of care are conducted in collaboration with the team of professionals, usually multidisciplinary, involved with the patient, and the plan of care is agreed in this context. The care co-ordinator then maintains the key relationship with the patient and co-ordinates their access to other professionals and specialists for specific interventions. This allows the patient to maintain their connection to the mental health services through a key relationship with one individual, rather than through a confusing array of titles and roles. It also allows an identified person (the care co-ordinator) to keep track of what care has been provided to the patient and any omissions or failures in the system. The care co-ordinator also manages the process of evaluating and reviewing the progress of care by arranging multidisciplinary CPA review meetings at the agreed time points. They collect information about the patient's care and progress from the different professionals involved, and collate this information so that it can easily be understood in the meeting. It is important to ensure that the care co-ordinator is well prepared and well supported in their role, as they carry a considerable burden of responsibility for the patient's care.

The nursing team

The nursing team is usually the largest and includes registered nurses as well as students and health care assistants who are not nurses but tend to be managed by nurses. Patients are entitled to know which nurse is responsible for providing their care at any given time (see Box 10.3).

Nursing teams vary in the way they structure the nurse's responsibilities and operate the 'named nurse' role in inpatient settings. There are three basic systems available: primary nursing; team nursing and the keyworker system. However, many teams use combinations or variations on these (see Figure 10.2).

Person

It is important to find the right person to whom to delegate the work. Ideally, this will be someone who has done the job before. You will need to assess whether they are qualified and able to perform the task and their level of proficiency. It is not always the case that work is delegated to people less experienced than oneself. However, when the other person does not have much experience, it is likely that they will take longer to complete the work. You may also find that, if you do not give very specific instructions, they may omit some parts of the work. For example, an instruction to 'help Mrs Brown with her lunch' may be taken literally and not include all the stages outlined above. Essentially, the other person needs to know and agree what it is they are being asked to do and when they are expected to have completed the work.

If you are delegated a task by a colleague, you need to satisfy yourself that you know what is expected of you and that you are competent to perform the task. You should not accept a task for which you are not competent (Nursing and Midwifery Council 2004).

SYSTEMS FOR MANAGING CARE

Managing care is also about how the care you deliver is organized. This requires having a systematic approach or framework within which to structure the work you are doing. There are several different frameworks for organizing individual care, for example Egan's (2002) 'systematic approach to effective helping', but the one that is most commonly used by nurses, and has been developed specifically for nurses, is known as 'the nursing process'.

The nursing process

There are several comprehensive texts on the nursing process in mental health nursing (see McFarland & Darand-Thomas 1990, Ward 2005). In brief, the nursing process is a problem-solving model with four stages that overlap and follow on from each other (see Figure 10.3).

As a student nurse, you are learning to provide care that meets the care needs of your patients. It is important to do this within a systematic structure so that the relationship between the patient's needs and the care you deliver is transparent. It is also important to make sure that this care can be carried on when you are not on duty and another nurse is providing the direct care to a patient. If you are working in the community or another setting where you have your own caseload of patients, there will be occasions when you

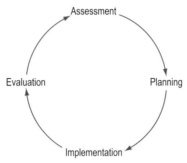

Figure 10.3 The nursing process: a cyclical model.

are on leave or unavailable for some other reason. Therefore, it is important that information about the patient's needs and their care plans are accurately documented. This is also a requirement of the Nursing and Midwifery Council (2002).

Assessment

It is important to gather as much information as possible about patients, their symptoms and how these affect their lives. The patient's abilities and needs are explored in depth to provide a clear picture of what their current needs are and how they affect the patient. This involves gathering information from a number of sources, including the patient themselves and those close to them and the medical and nursing notes. A clear statement of these needs is agreed between the nurse and the patient. The statement of need has three components: the underlying reason why the need is unmet; the unmet need itself; and the effect the unmet need has on the patient's life (Box 10.5).

Planning and goal setting

The planning stage is where the action required to meet the patient's needs is identified. This involves setting a long-term objective, outlining the ultimate aim of the care and several shorter term goals, which serve as manageable 'staging posts' towards the longer term objective. Identifying goals usually

---

Box 10.5 Example of a statement of a patient's need

Because of self-doubt associated with feelings of worthlessness, Henry finds it difficult to establish and maintain social relationships. This leads to him spending most of his time on his own and feeling lonely.

Box 10.6 'SMART' acronym for objectives and goals

S – specific: a concise statement of the desired outcome

M – measurable: it is easy to distinguish when the objective or goal has been completed and when it has not

A – achievable: it is possible to complete the objective or goal

R – realistic: given all the circumstances and people involved, it is reasonable to expect that the objective or goal can be carried out within the timeframe

T – time oriented: a point in time by which the objective or goal will be completed is included.

---

means making explicit what action each person involved (patient, nurse, carers, other professionals or agencies) is expected to take to contribute to meeting the objective. The objective and goals need to be stated in a form that allows a clear evaluation of whether they have been achieved. One possibility is using the acronym 'SMART' (see Box 10.6) to assist in the writing of objectives and goals.

The objectives and goals are negotiated between the patient and nurse. What is expected of the patient, the nurse, the carers and of any other professionals involved should all be clearly identified in a document called a 'care plan'. The timescale is also agreed and includes setting a realistic date to review the progress of the care. Each person, particularly the patient, should keep a copy of this document so they know what is expected of them.

Implementation

In the implementation stage, the care that was agreed in the planning stage is delivered. Each person performs the action they were allocated and agreed in the care plan. Using the example in Box 10.7 (overleaf), Henry should be clear about what it is that he has agreed to do (this includes joining a club and starting conversations). The work for John (the student nurse) is to meet with Henry and monitor his progress at each stage (identifying a social setting, joining and starting conversations).

Evaluation

The evaluation stage comes at the end of the process but, because the nursing process is cyclical, the evaluation stage leads back into a new assessment. The evaluation involves a review of the care that has been delivered during the implementation phase to see whether the goals are being achieved, if these

> ## Box 10.7 Examples of objectives and goals
>
> *Objective*
> Within the next 6 months, Henry will establish social relationships with two people.
>
> *Goals*
> Within the next week, Henry and John (student nurse) will identify two social settings that Henry is interested in joining, e.g. club, gym, evening class.
>
> Within 1 month, Henry will have joined the two social settings identified.
>
> Within 1 week of joining each club, gym or evening class, Henry will start a social conversation with at least one other person.
>
> Each subsequent week of membership, Henry will engage in a social conversation with at least one person he has spoken to before, and start a social conversation with at least one new person.

are contributing to achievement of the objective and if these are helping to meet the patient's needs. In the example, this would include reviewing whether Henry had:

- identified two social settings
- joined or taken up membership of the two settings
- in the first week of joining, started a conversation with one person
- in the subsequent weeks, continued conversing with the same person and begun a conversation with one new person.

There may be several reasons why the objectives and goals have not been met, or why the planned care does not meet the patient's needs; it may be because the needs that were targeted were not the main needs and that these have not been addressed. Or there may be aspects of need that were not clearly identified during the assessment stage. For example, Henry may have joined a club or evening class but may not have spoken to anyone. Sometimes, one of the people assigned a role in the planning stage has not performed this adequately, and often this is because the expectation was unrealistic. Sometimes, patients have unrealistic expectations of themselves, and they can learn useful lessons about their care needs through an unachieved objective. Alternatively, it may be that there has been a change in the patient's condition and so their needs have changed. All these possibilities require a reassessment of the patient's needs and a new plan for care. For example, it may have become clear that Henry's difficulties in starting a conversation were due to high levels of anxiety or because he didn't know how to start a conversation. The evaluation then leads to identifying new goals.

Theoretical models

The nursing process is usually used in conjunction with a theoretical or conceptual model (see also Chapter 7, Assessment). A number of theoretical models drawn from nursing, medicine and psychology are available. They provide a structure for the assessment, describe the role of the nurse or other professional in providing care and indicate the type of interventions that are appropriate.

One such model that is commonly used by nurses is that of Peplau (1952) (see also Chapter 2). According to Peplau's model, assessment is concerned with the patient's ability to meet their own needs from a broad list of 10 universal human 'felt needs'. Peplau (1952) sees the key intervention as the relationship between the nurse and the patient.

Different theoretical models may be used according to the clinical setting or the focus of the service (Tyrer & Steinberg 2005). They may focus more directly on the pattern of the patient's symptoms or on their ability to function socially. Alternatively, psychological models can also be used, which focus either on the psychodynamics of the patient's subjective experience or on their thinking and behaviour (cognitive behavioural models). As a student, you will work in a range of settings where the work is structured in different ways according to the different frameworks and models in use.

COMMUNICATION IN DIFFERENT CONTEXTS

In Figure 10.1, we identified different contexts in which care is managed; these are individual, team and delegation. The reality is that these are not separate contexts but all part of the practice environment that includes the patient, the student and the staff team.

The student has to learn how to communicate (or pass on information) in a way that is appropriate to each context. In the individual context, information is initially exchanged between patient and student. However, the student also has to communicate to the registered nurse exactly what happened. Students, especially in inpatient settings, can spend a lot of time with patients and therefore have access to large amounts of information (see Box 10.8).

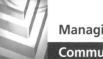
> **Box 10.8 Communication in different contexts**
>
> Imagine that you are in the dayroom with a patient who starts to talk about a TV programme you both watched and enjoyed. You discuss this for about 10 minutes.
>
> Think about how you might report this conversation to staff in different contexts, e.g. mentor, handover, ward round.

You could begin by thinking about the different contexts in which this conversation might be reported and the goal of the context. The first context could be the student meeting their mentor. Here, the primary goal is for the student to learn about managing the care they deliver. In this instance, a verbatim (word for word) account of the conversation may be useful and could be accompanied by a verbal report about what you observed about the patient and yourself. Reflecting on the conversation might include trying to clarify the purpose of the conversation as well as thinking about whether a different type of interaction would have been more useful. Through this type of discussion, the student can learn how to deliver care. In addition, the student can begin to understand that, in mental health nursing, which is essentially an interpersonal discipline, much of the learning is about how to manage ourselves.

In the mentor context, the student can also be helped to identify how information obtained in one context (individual) can be transferred into another context (team) such as a care programme approach (CPA) meeting, ward round or staff handover. Here, such a detailed account would not help to support the work of the context (that is to make decisions about the patient's care), although summarizing the key points would be helpful. So, in this context, some type of filter is necessary; the difficulty for students is often identifying what information to include and what to leave out.

In practice, most students will be strongly influenced by how they see other staff behaving and will try to conform to the norm of the environment that they are in. For example, if the staff team usually focuses on information about the patient or service user's strengths or abilities, the student will do so too. In relation to the example in Box 10.8, this might include reporting that the patient was able to concentrate on a TV programme that lasted for 1 hour and then discuss some of the main issues. Here, the student is presenting a summary of what they observed in relation to the patient's speech (see Chapter 3, Observation). As the student becomes more knowledgeable, they will begin to see that data that is in some respects quite descriptive can also provide information about aspects of functioning such as concentration and memory.

Key time points

Although it is always important to take care regarding the exchange of information, there are certain times when it is useful to be even more vigilant. These are times of transition when patients (or staff) are moving from one setting or state to another. A common example involving inpatients relates to admission and discharge. For some patients, admission to hospital will be unplanned or will involve little or no time to prepare, regardless of whether it involves being admitted informally or under a section of the Mental Health Act (HMSO 1983). This may mean leaving behind people for whom the patient is the main carer, including children, parents or other relatives, as well as pets. There may be serious problems at home that need attention, such as leaking pipes, as well as key appointments, perhaps regarding housing or benefits. Any or all of these issues may cause considerable anxiety at a time that is already stressful.

A thorough assessment should identify these issues as well as similarly relevant information at the point of discharge (for example, the patient is due to be discharged, but it is winter and they do not have any heating). Being sensitive to the patient's concerns about home may help to identify these issues at an early point. Although, as a student, it is not your responsibility to identify these issues, you may become aware of them because of the amount of time you spend with the patient. Your responsibility is to ensure that the information is passed to the staff team.

It is helpful to be aware that these transition times are points at which it is easy for information to be lost because staff have forgotten to pass on what they know. It would be a rare student who has never had the experience of leaving the practice environment and suddenly thinking 'I forgot to tell x . . .'. This is where 'formal' spaces for reporting, such as the shift handover and care programme approach (CPA) meetings, are very useful, as listening to another nurse or other professional speaking about the patient can often help to jog one's own memory for information that might otherwise be forgotten. Along with managing time, students must learn how to feed back information from the patient to the staff team and vice versa within reasonable time limits.

Rules of reporting

The student can operate a simple rule here: any information they receive that has implications for the patient's physical or psychological safety must be reported immediately to a registered nurse (or the nurse in charge). This rule also applies if you remember something once you have left the practice environment – you must telephone to inform the nurse in charge straight away. If you are in any doubt about whether the information you have has any implications for the patient's safety, then it is preferable to err on the side of caution and telephone. When you next meet your mentor or tutor, you can explore whether it was necessary to telephone with the information.

MANAGING CARE AND THE ESSENTIAL SKILLS

The essential skills of developing a therapeutic relationship, observation, taking on different roles and reflection provide the building blocks for delivering care, and they provide information that contributes to the management of care. Managing care is about both delivering care and being able to see 'the bigger picture'. This includes getting feedback from the patient or service user about their experience of the care they are receiving. It is also necessary to make ongoing evaluations regarding the efficacy of care.

Information that is obtained through a therapeutic relationship and your own observations will be used by nurses and the multidisciplinary team to inform care management discussions. As you take on additional responsibilities, you should pay attention to your emotional reactions. For example, as you move from observing to participating in discussions about managing care, some people will notice that they feel excited about taking on a new role, whereas others will feel apprehensive. You can use the tool of reflection to learn about how care is managed, whether this is care you are delivering directly or whether you focus on how the nurse in charge delegates work to others.

SUMMARY

- There are different contexts in which care has to be managed, and each context will have its own goals.
- In the individual context, the emphasis is on structuring meetings and managing time.
- Nurses work within a multidisciplinary team.
- Nursing teams use systems to manage care, such as primary or team nursing or the key worker system.
- Effective delegation involves a match between the task and the person best able to complete it.
- Nurses hold a key position in managing multidisciplinary communication.

References

Burns T (2004) *Community Mental Health Teams. A Guide to Current Practices.* Oxford: Oxford University Press.

Department of Health (1999) *Effective Care Co-ordination in Mental Health Services: Modernising the CPA.* London: Department of Health.

Egan G (2002) *The Skilled Helper: Problem-Management and Opportunity Development Approach to Helping,* 7th edn. Pacific Grove, CA: Brooks/Cole Publishing.

HMSO (1983) Mental Health Act. London: HMSO.

McFarland G, Darand-Thomas M (1990) *Psychiatric Mental Health Nursing: The Application of the Nursing Process.* Philadelphia, PA: Lippincott, Williams and Wilkins.

Nursing and Midwifery Council (2002) *An NMC Guide for Students of Nursing and Midwifery.* London: NMC.

Nursing and Midwifery Council (2004) *Code of Professional Conduct: Standards for Conduct, Performance and Ethics.* London: NMC.

Onyett S (2004) Functional teams and whole systems. In: I Norman and I Ryrie (eds) *The Art and Science of Mental Health Nursing. A Textbook of Principles and Practice.* Maidenhead: Open University Press.

Peplau H (1952) *Interpersonal Relations in Nursing.* New York: GP Putnam.

Ritchie JH (1994) *The Report of the Enquiry into the Care and Treatment of Christopher Clunis Presented to the Chairman of the North East Thames and South East Thames Regional Health Authorities.* London: HMSO.

Tyrer P, Steinberg D (2005) *Models for Mental Disorder,* 4th edn. Chichester: Wiley.

Ward M (2005) The nursing process in UK mental health care: application to a field. In: Habermann M (ed) *The Nursing Process: A Global Concept.* London: Churchill Livingstone.

Appendix

Clinical observation skills

The following skills have been reproduced, with kind permission, from Nicol et al. (2004):

- temperature recording
- pulse recording
- counting respirations
- blood pressure recording
- weighing the patient
- blood glucose monitoring
- urinalysis.

Temperature recording

Preparation

Patient
- Explain procedure, to gain consent and co-operation.
- Assess patient regarding suitable site for temperature recording.
- Patient should not have had a hot drink, smoked a cigarette or exercised within the previous 15 minutes.

Equipment/environment
- Disposable chemical thermometer, e.g. TempaDot.
- Observation chart.

Nurse
- Hands must be clean.

Procedure

Oral
1. Ask the patient to open their mouth, and gently insert the thermometer under their tongue, next to the frenulum. This is adjacent to a large artery (sublingual artery), so the temperature will be close to core temperature (Figure A.1a).
2. Ask the patient to close their lips, but not their teeth, around the thermometer to prevent cool air circulating in the mouth.
3. Leave in position for the recommended length of time (usually 1 minute).
4. Remove the thermometer, taking care not to touch the part that has been in the patient's mouth. In accordance with the manufacturer's instructions, read the temperature by noting the way that the dots have changed colour (see Figure A.1c).

A

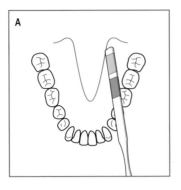

B

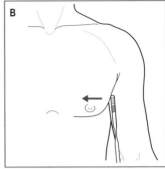

C

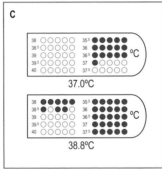

Figure A.1 Disposable chemical thermometer. (a) Positioning the thermometer for oral use. (b) Positioning the thermometer for axillary use. (c) Reading the thermometer (from Nicol et al 2000, with permission from Elsevier).

Axilla

1. Ask/assist the patient to expose their axilla. For an accurate recording, the axilla must be dry.
2. With the dots facing the chest wall, position the thermometer vertically between the arm and the chest wall and ask/assist the patient to keep their arm close against the chest to ensure good contact with the skin (see Figure A.1b).
3. Leave in position for the recommended length of time (usually 3 minutes).
4. In accordance with the manufacturer's instructions, read the temperature by noting the way that the dots have changed colour (see Figure A.1c).

Post procedure

Patient

- Ensure patient comfort.
- Answer any questions regarding the recording.

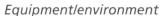

Equipment/environment
- Dispose of the thermometer into the clinical waste bag.

Nurse
- Chart temperature recording.
- Report any abnormality.

Points for practice

1. If the patient is unconscious, confused, prone to seizures, has mouth sores or has undergone oral surgery, the oral site should not be used for temperature measurement.
2. The rectal site is no longer recommended except when an electronic probe is being used.
3. Mercury thermometers are no longer widely used as there are risks of breakage. If a mercury thermometer is used, it must be cleaned before and after use, and the mercury must be shaken down to the bottom of the scale before use.
4. The normal range for temperature is between 36°C and 37.2°C.
5. Electronic oral and tympanic thermometers are increasingly being used; the technique for these is described below.

Using electronic thermometers

Oral

Electronic oral thermometers are increasingly being used in hospitals. They are efficient, quick and easy to use, with an audible signal indicating when the maximum temperature has been reached. The probe, covered by a disposable plastic cover, is placed under the tongue in the same way as a disposable thermometer (Figure A.2). Each cover is for use by one patient only and is usually kept clean and dry on the patient's locker between uses. It is discarded when the patient is discharged from the ward.

Tympanic

Some electronic thermometers are designed to measure the temperature by inserting a probe into the outer ear, adjacent to (but not touching) the tympanic membrane (Figure A.3). An infrared light detects heat radiated from the tympanic membrane and provides a digital reading. This usually takes only a few seconds, and an audible signal indicates when the reading is complete. This provides a more accurate measure of body core temperature as it is close to the carotid artery. A special cover is used for each patient to prevent cross-infection. The patient may need more explanation than usual because,

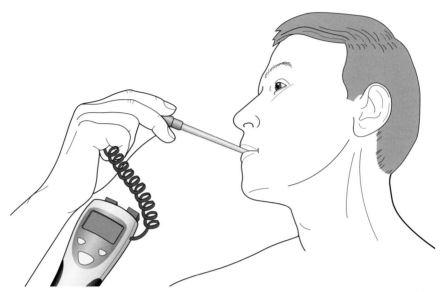

Figure A.2 Oral electronic thermometer (from Nicol et al 2000, with permission from Elsevier).

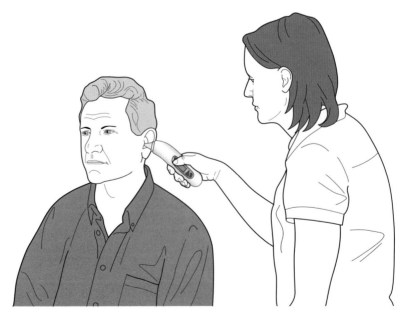

Figure A.3 Tympanic membrane thermometer (from Nicol et al 2000, with permission from Elsevier).

although most people will have had their temperature recorded at some point, they may be surprised to find you approaching their ear! It is a simple technique, but any of the following may lead to an inaccurate reading: wax in the ear; a cracked or dirty lens; poor fitting in the ear; and if the patient has been recently lying on the ear that is used (Jevon 2001).

Pulse recording

Preparation

Patient
- Explain the procedure, to gain consent and co-operation.
- The patient should be resting, either lying down or sitting. Allow time to rest after physical activity, emotional upset or smoking.

Equipment/environment
- A watch with a second hand.
- Observation chart.

Nurse
- No special preparation is necessary unless required by the patient's condition, e.g. methicillin-resistant *Staphylococcus aureus* (MRSA).

Procedure

1. Choose a site to record the pulse. For most routine recordings, the radial pulse is used (Figure A.4).
2. Using your first and second fingers to feel the pulse; lightly but firmly compress the artery.
3. Count the number of beats for 1 minute. If the pulse is regular, it is sufficient to count for 30 seconds and double the result. If the pulse is irregular, count for a full minute. The normal range is 60–80 beats per minute.
4. In addition to the rate per minute, note the rhythm, i.e. whether it is regular or irregular, and the volume/strength of the pulse felt.
5. Note the colour of the patient's skin and mucous membranes (inside lower eyelid). Pallor may indicate anaemia, while a bluish colour indicates a lack of oxygen (cyanosis). In dark-skinned patients, it is easier to detect this in the nail beds.

Post procedure

Patient
- Explain the results and discuss the reasons for any changes in care.

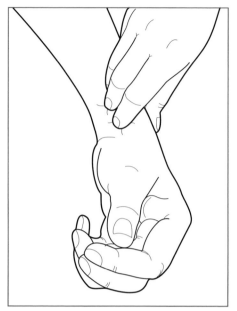

Figure A.4 Taking the radial pulse (from Nicol et al 2000, with permission from Elsevier).

Nurse
- Record the findings and report any abnormalities.

Points for practice

1. The usual site for recording the pulse rate is at the wrist, where the radial pulse is easily felt.
2. Pulses may also be felt at other sites, e.g. in the carotid artery in the neck; this site is used when a person collapses suddenly as the radial pulse would not be appropriate.

Counting respirations

Preparation

Patient
- The patient should be relaxed and resting, or recent activity should be noted.
- Do not inform the patient when you will be assessing breathing.

Equipment/environment
- Watch with a second hand.

Nurse
- The hands should be clean.

Procedure

1. Observe the movement of the chest wall and count the respirations for 60 seconds.
2. Observe the rhythm and depth of respirations.
3. Observe the patient's colour for signs of cyanosis.
4. Observe for symmetry of chest movement and whether accessory muscles are being used.
5. Observe for the following:
   - difficulty in breathing
   - pain on breathing and its location
   - noisy respiration – whether there is wheezing or other unusual sounds
   - cough – whether dry or productive
   - sputum – amount, colour and consistency.

Post procedure

Patient
- Ensure the patient is comfortable. A patient with breathing difficulties may be most comfortable sitting upright.

Nurse
- Record the respiratory observations and report any abnormalities.
- Adjust the frequency of observations as necessary.

Points for practice

1. A more accurate observation is obtained if the patient is unaware that their respirations are being counted. Many nurses achieve this by pretending to be feeling the radial pulse when in fact observing the movement of the chest wall (Figure A.5).
2. If breathing is very shallow and difficult to observe, lightly rest your hand on the patient's chest or abdomen to feel movement. The normal rate for an adult is 12–20 breaths per minute.
3. Cyanosis is a blue discoloration of the skin and mucous membranes and is most noticeable around the lips, earlobes, mouth and fingertips. In dark-skinned patients, signs of poor perfusion or cyanosis may be detected if the area around the lips or nail beds is dusky in colour.

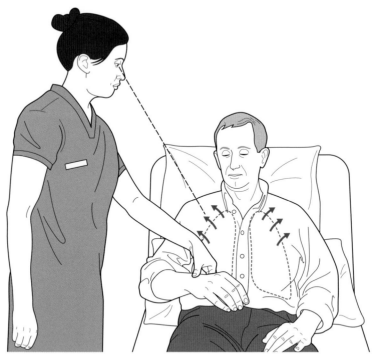

Figure A.5 Monitoring the respiration rate while apparently counting the pulse (from Nicol et al 2000, with permission from Elsevier).

Blood pressure recording

Preparation

Patient
- Explain the procedure, to gain consent and co-operation.
- The patient should be resting in a bed, couch or chair, in a quiet location, with their legs uncrossed.
- The patient should not have had a meal, alcohol or caffeine or have smoked or exercised in the previous 30 minutes.

Equipment/environment
- Sphygmomanometer with appropriate size cuff (PFP 1 and 2).
- Stethoscope.
- Alcohol-impregnated swabs.
- Observation chart.

Nurse

- The hands should be clean.
- No special preparation is necessary unless required by the patient's condition, e.g. MRSA.

Procedure

1. Assess the patient's knowledge of the procedure and explain as necessary.
2. Ensure the patient is resting in a comfortable position. If a comparison between lying and standing blood pressure is required, the 'lying' recording should be done first.
3. When applying the cuff, no clothing should be underneath it. If clothing constricts the arm, remove the arm from the sleeve (PFP 3).
4. Apply the cuff such that the centre of the 'bladder' is over the brachial artery, 2–3 cm above the antecubital fossa (PFP 4).
5. The arm should be positioned so that the cuff is level with the heart and may be more comfortable resting on a pillow.
6. The sphygmomanometer should be placed on a firm surface, with the dial clearly visible.
7. Perform a radial check to estimate systolic blood pressure (Figure A.6) (PFP 5). Locate the radial pulse. Squeeze the bulb slowly to inflate the cuff while still feeling the pulse. Observe the dial and note the level when the pulse can no longer be felt. Open the valve fully to quickly release the pressure in the cuff.
8. If using a communal stethoscope, clean the earpieces with an alcohol-impregnated swab. Curving the ends of the stethoscope slightly forward, place the earpieces in your ears. Check that the tubes are not twisted.
9. Check that the stethoscope is turned to the diaphragm side by tapping it with your finger.
10. Palpate the brachial artery, which is located on the medial aspect of the antecubital fossa (just to the side of the midline, on the side nearest to the patient).
11. Place the diaphragm of the stethoscope over the artery, and hold it in place with your thumb while your fingers support the patient's elbow (Figure A.7).
12. Position yourself so that the dial of the sphygmomanometer is clearly visible.
13. Ensure that the valve on the bulb is closed and inflate the cuff to 20–30 mmHg above the level noted in step 7. Open the valve to allow the needle of the dial to drop slowly (2 mm per second).

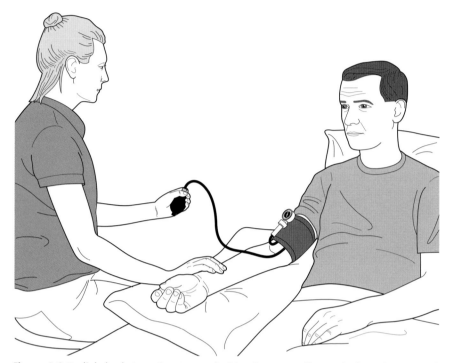

Figure A.6 Radial check to estimate systolic blood pressure (from Nicol et al 2000, with permission from Elsevier).

14. While observing the needle of the dial as it falls, listen for Korotkoff (thudding) sounds:
    - the *systolic* pressure is the level at which these are first heard.
    - the *diastolic* pressure is the level at which the sounds disappear.
15. Once the sounds have disappeared, open the valve fully to completely deflate the cuff, and remove it from the patient's arm.
16. If a lying and standing blood pressure is required, do not remove the cuff. Ask the patient to stand and then repeat steps 10–15 of the procedure (PFP 6).

Post procedure

Patient
- Replace clothing and ensure the patient is comfortable.

Equipment/environment
- Replace equipment.
- Clean the earpieces of the stethoscope.

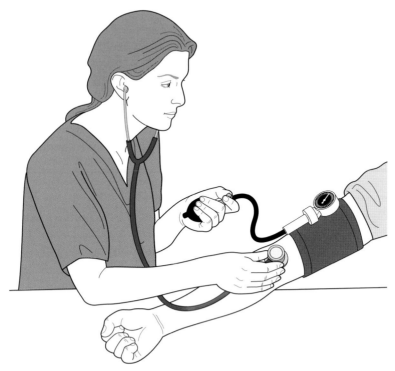

Figure A.7 Stethoscope over the brachial artery (from Nicol et al 2000, with permission from Elsevier).

Nurse

- Chart the blood pressure accurately. Report any variation from previous recordings.

Points for practice

1. The sphygmomanometer may be an aneroid or a mercury type. These are used in exactly the same way except that a column of mercury, which must be placed in an upright position, is observed instead of a dial. Because mercury releases dangerous fumes if spilt, aneroid sphygmomanometers are replacing the mercury type. Electronic blood pressure recording machines are now often used. The cuff should be positioned in the same way as described in step 4, but no stethoscope is required because the machine provides a digital display of the systolic and diastolic pressures.
2. The bladder inside the cuff must cover at least 80% of the circumference of the upper arm.

3. If the patient is receiving intravenous therapy, avoid using the arm that has the intravenous cannula or infusion in progress.
4. If the patient is unable to lift their arm, tuck the patient's hand under your arm to support the arm while you position the cuff.
5. The radial check allows you to estimate the systolic blood pressure and avoid inflating the cuff unnecessarily high during step 13. This can be performed while palpating the brachial artery instead. If using an electronic blood pressure machine, steps 7–15 are not necessary; simply press the start button and the machine will inflate itself and then display the systolic and diastolic pressures.
6. If recording lying and standing blood pressure, do not remove the cuff between recordings, keep it in the same position. The doctor may have requested that the patient is standing for at least 5 minutes before the standing blood pressure is recorded. Be aware that the patient may feel dizzy on getting out of bed (postural hypotension).

Weighing patients and service users

Preparation

Patient
- Encourage the patient to empty their bladder.
- Weigh the person on the same scales, at the same time each day/week and in similar clothing (PFP 1).

Equipment/environment
- The scales must be on a level surface.
- Use the same scales for regular weighing.
- Ensure the pointer is at zero or weights are to the left, at zero.

Nurse
- An apron should be worn if the person requires assistance.

Procedure

1. Position the scales for easy access and apply the brakes.
2. Ask/assist the person to sit on the scales or stand on the platform. If electronic scales are being used, plug them into the mains before the person steps on or sits down.
3. If sitting, ensure that the person's feet are off the floor.
4. Ask the person to remain still while you note the reading.
5. If the scales are manual, check the person's previous weight to determine the approximate position and move the heavier weight bar (kilograms) to

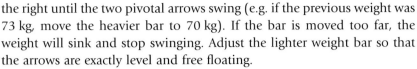

the right until the two pivotal arrows swing (e.g. if the previous weight was 73 kg, move the heavier bar to 70 kg). If the bar is moved too far, the weight will sink and stop swinging. Adjust the lighter weight bar so that the arrows are exactly level and free floating.

6. Note the reading by adding the position of the heavier bar (e.g. 70 kg) to that of the lighter bar (e.g. 3.5 kg; total equals 73.5 kg).

7. If the weight is very different from a recent previous weight, check it again and, if confirmed, report it.

Post procedure

Patient
- Assist the person to replace clothing/shoes, etc. as necessary.

Equipment/environment
- Return the scales to their storage place and clean if necessary.

Nurse
- Document weight and report any unexpected loss or gain.

Points for practice

1. It is important to use the same scales each time as most scales will give a slightly different weight. When weighing patients and service users regularly, what is important is what is happening to the weight; whether is it going up, going down or staying the same. Only by using the same set of scales will such comparisons be accurate. Our weight changes throughout the day, and so it is also important to weigh people at the same time of day and to ensure that they are wearing similar clothing. The type of clothing worn (e.g. whether a jacket and shoes were worn) should be noted with the weight.

Blood glucose monitoring

Preparation

Patient
- Explain the procedure, to gain consent and co-operation.
- Ensure the patient's hands are clean. Do not use alcohol wipes (PFP 1).
- Ask the patient to choose the finger to be used for the procedure.

Equipment/environment
- Glucose meter.
- Finger-pricking device or lancet (PFP 2).

- Gauze swab/cotton-wool ball, according to local policy.
- Blood glucose testing strips.

Nurse
- Wash and dry hands thoroughly.
- Put on gloves.

Procedure

1. Ensure all equipment is within easy reach and the patient is comfortable.
2. If necessary, assist the patient with washing and drying of the finger/ hand.
3. Use new lancets and platforms (if finger-pricking device used) for each test (PFP 2).
4. Check the expiry date of the testing strips, prepare the glucose meter and insert the testing strip according to the manufacturer's instructions (PFP 3).
5. Using the appropriate device, prick the side of the patient's fingertip, avoiding the thumbs, index and little fingers where possible (PFP 4).
6. Allow a drop of blood to fall onto the testing strip – do not smear (PFP 5).
7. Ask the patient to press on the site, using the gauze swab/cotton-wool ball, to stem bleeding and reduce the risk of bruising.
8. Wait for the meter to provide a digital display of the result (PFP 6).

Post procedure

Patient
- Ensure the patient is comfortable.
- Ensure bleeding has stopped.

Equipment/environment
- Dispose of all sharps and contaminated waste in the appropriate containers.
- Return equipment as appropriate.

Nurse
- Remove gloves and wash hands.
- Document the result and report any abnormalities.

Points for practice

1. The patient's hands must be clean. If there is any possibility that there may have been contact with substances such as fruit juice, the finger should be

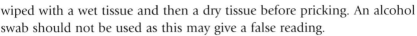

wiped with a wet tissue and then a dry tissue before pricking. An alcohol swab should not be used as this may give a false reading.

2. Where possible use a finger-pricking device, as it is more likely to ensure a good blood flow and is less painful. Before pricking the patient's finger, hold the hand downwards to encourage blood flow, and make a light tourniquet with your hand around the finger to ensure that sufficient blood is present in the tip of the finger. Avoid 'milking' blood into the finger as the local blood composition may be disturbed by intermingling with tissue fluid. Taking time to encourage blood flow before pricking the finger will reduce the need for pricking again, which can be distressing for the patient.

3. Preparation of the glucose meter usually involves checking that it has been calibrated for the particular batch of testing strips that are being used.

4. Blood glucose monitoring can be painful for the patient, especially if performed several times a day. Non-invasive methods of measuring blood glucose levels (e.g. Glucowatch™) are currently being developed.

5. The drop of blood should fall on to the strip rather than be 'wiped on', as this may lead to an inaccurate result.

6. With some glucose meters, the strip is inserted into the meter after the blood is dropped on to it. Follow the manufacturer's instructions regarding timing and wiping prior to insertion into the machine.

Urinalysis

Preparation

Patient
- Ask the patient to provide a urine specimen or obtain a specimen, e.g. catheter specimen (PFP 1).

Equipment/environment
- Fresh urine specimen in clean container/jug.
- Urine reagent sticks.
- Watch with a second hand.

Nurse
- The hands should be clean and gloves should be worn.
- An apron should be worn if there is a risk of splashing.

Procedure

1. Check the expiry date of the reagent sticks and make sure that you are familiar with the manufacturer's instructions for use.

2. Remove a stick, making sure that you do not touch the coloured reagent pads with your hands. Replace the lid (PFP 2).
3. Dip the stick into the urine so that the reagent pads are completely immersed. Tap the stick against the side of the container/jug to remove excess urine (PFP 3).
4. Note the time on your watch. Accurate timing according to the manufacturer's instructions is crucial.
5. When the correct period of time has elapsed, read off the results by holding the stick alongside (but not touching) the pot and comparing the colour of each reagent pad with those displayed on the side (Figure A.8). Make a mental note of the results.

Urine reagent sticks commonly test for the following:

1. Specific gravity (how concentrated or dilute the urine is – normal range 1005–1030).
2. pH (the acidity or alkalinity of the urine – normal range 4.5–8.0).
3. Protein, glucose, ketones, blood and bilirubin. All these are negative in normal urine. The presence of these abnormalities might indicate the following (Baillie 2001):
   - Protein (proteinuria) – urinary tract infection.
   - Glucose (glycosuria) – diabetes mellitus or sometimes in pregnancy.
   - Ketones (ketonuria) – excessive fat metabolism due to diabetic ketoacidosis, vomiting or severe dieting.

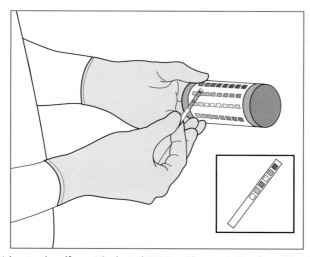

Figure A.8 Urine testing (from Nicol et al 2000, with permission from Elsevier).

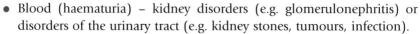

- Blood (haematuria) – kidney disorders (e.g. glomerulonephritis) or disorders of the urinary tract (e.g. kidney stones, tumours, infection).
- Bilirubin – liver disease (e.g. hepatitis) or biliary tract obstruction (e.g. gallstones, carcinoma of the head of pancreas).

Post procedure

Patient
- Discuss the result with the patient as appropriate.

Equipment/environment
- Discard the used stick in the clinical waste and dispose of the urine safely.
- Clean or dispose of the container/jug according to local policy.

Nurse
- Remove gloves and wash hands.
- Document urinalysis and report any abnormalities.

Points for practice

1. The urine specimen should be fresh, ideally less than 30 minutes old.
2. The lid of the reagent sticks pot must always be replaced immediately after use to prevent moisture getting in.
3. Removing excess urine prevents the urine running from each reagent pad into the others and contaminating the result.
4. Make a mental note of the results or, if necessary, jot them down on a piece of paper. Do not take the patient's charts into the dirty utility/sluice room, to prevent contamination or splashing with water.

Recommended reading for further information

Baillie L (2001) *Developing Practical Nursing Skills*. London: Arnold.

Blows WT (2001) *The Biological Basis of Nursing: Clinical Observations*. London: Routledge.

Burden M (2001) Diabetes: blood glucose monitoring. *Nursing Times* 97 (8), 36–39.

Esmond G (2001) *Respiratory Nursing*. Edinburgh: Baillière Tindall.

Jevon P (2001) Using a tympanic thermometer. *Nursing Times* 97 (9), 43–44.

Nicol M, Bavin C, Bedford-Turner S, Cronin P, Rawlings-Anderson K (2004) *Essential Nursing Skills*, 2nd edn. Edinburgh: Mosby.

Skinner S (2006) *Understanding Clinical Investigations*, 2nd edn. Edinburgh: Baillière Tindall.

Index

Note

Page numbers in *italics* refer to figures, tables and boxes.